# Queen Jin's
# Handbook
# of Pregnancy

We are so excited for
you guys !!
Just a cute book
for some fun reading

♡ Mary + Jon
+
Noah

# Queen Jin's Handbook of Pregnancy

## Fred Jeremy Seligson

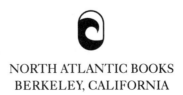

NORTH ATLANTIC BOOKS
BERKELEY, CALIFORNIA

Published by
North Atlantic Books
P.O. Box 12327
Berkeley, California 94712

Circular illustrations by Han Yoon-Ki
Cover and book design by Jennifer Dunn

Printed in the United States of America

Cover painting "Woman Applying Cosmetics Before a Mirror" by Kim Hong Do (1745–1814), courtesy of Seoul National University Museum.

*Queen Jin's Handbook of Pregnancy* is sponsored by the Society for the Study of Native Arts and Sciences, a nonprofit educational corporation whose goals are to develop an educational and crosscultural perspective linking various scientific, social, and artistic fields; to nurture a holistic view of arts, sciences, humanities, and healing; and to publish and distribute literature on the relationship of mind, body, and nature.

This book is a sharing of ideas and not a doctor's prescription. It should be accepted only as long as the mother, the primary guide, feels it is doing herself and her baby some good, but the responsibility must be hers. She should always consult a medical doctor or an Oriental Medical Doctor (O.M.D.) with any questions.

---

North Atlantic Books are available through most bookstores. To contact North Atlantic directly, call 800-337-2665 or visit our website at www.northatlanticbooks.com.

Substantial discounts on bulk quantities of North Atlantic books are available to corporations, professional associations, and other organizations. For details and discount information, contact the special sales department at North Atlantic Books.

---

Library of Congress Cataloging-in-Publication Data

Seligson, Fred Jeremy.
   Queen Jin's handbook of pregnancy / by Fred Jeremy Seligson.
      p.  cm.
     ISBN 1-55643-405-7 (alk. paper)
     1. Pregnancy—Asia—Miscellanea—Handbooks, manuals, etc. 2. Pregnancy—Asia—Cross-cultural studies—Handbooks, manuals, etc. I. Title.

  RG556.S30 2001
  618.2'4'095—dc21
                          2001030930

1  2  3  4  5  6  7  /  06  05  04  03  02

# A Gift for the Parents and Children
## of Our World

*Let us write the truth on a jade stone, and keep it in a gold box in the shrine where our descendants can see it.*

*They must know the reasons for, and preserve, these teachings for the womb.*

—Ja Hee, *The New Record* (130 B.C.)

*Shakily, hurrying down the twined, leafy vines of a beanstalk from above the clouds, carrying the "Secret of Existence"; dangling. I'm afraid of falling.*

*A bearded friend urges me on and, somehow, I drop to ground. We scramble off as a giantess flies over, just missing us, and lands prone on a soft, grassy bank nearby.*

*Looking back, she recognizes that we are not wrongdoers. Presently her robust husband and their graceful daughter appear. He wears a traditional Korean hemp shirt and baggy trousers, topped by a blue green vest; and she, an abundant, cherry pink silk dress; cheerful and at ease.*

According to my interpretation of this dream, the beanstalk is an umbilical cord connecting the nurturing Earth and Sky. The friend is my editor, David Kosofsky. The giant is Father Sky; the giantess, Mother Earth. Their daughter is also mine. Now "The Secret of Existence" is yours, too!

# Contents

# Foreword

This book, a love letter to the future parents and children of our world, is a cultural treasure artfully conjured from the heart of a poet and the mind of a scholar illuminating a high tradition of pregnancy and birth dating back to the twelfth century B.C. The timing of such a work is surely auspicious as Western obstetrics, yet in its infancy, threatens to engulf all previous visions of pregnancy in cultures past and present across the globe.

Based on three decades of living and teaching in Asia, and powerfully motivated by the adventure of two pregnancies with Young Im, his Korean wife, Seligson writes of an enchanting journey through time. Voices of oriental men and women speak to us of their daily lives and ideals for pregnancy and birth. Young Im and her ancestors teach us by their meditations and prayers, their letters, dreams (and dream interpretations), their foods, drinks and herbal formulas, their use of music and color, and in poems and proverbs. This material is chronologically grouped around three major epochs of parenting, first (notably) preparing for conception; second, nurturing the baby in the womb; and finally giving birth. Running through this tapestry is the unobtrusive thread of the writer's personal experiences.

Seligson tells how he fell in love with the idea of nurturing, with his wife, a healthy and compassionate child—inspired by the example and rules of Queen Jin, a woman of towering influence in China, Japan, and Korea for over 3,000 years. Her explosive contribution: *Embryonic Education*, a remarkably prescient set of guidelines for royals and aristocrats, for their servants, and eventually for the rest of humanity generation after generation. Her credibility was secured by the birth of her son, the sage-king Wan who wrote the classic *I-Ching*.

The timing of this book is auspicious also because of the burst of interest in prenatal medical and psychological research in the West over the last two decades and, most especially, the topic of prenatal stimulation. Amidst the traditional controversy over the possible value of such efforts by parents, experimental research has tipped the scale sharply in the affirmative by providing documentary evidence of its many salutary benefits.[1] The stage is therefore set, after fourteen centuries of widespread indifference, for the convergence of insight from the East and scientific verification from the West, allowing a full appreciation of the sentient nature of babies in the womb. This convergence bodes well for the future of the world.

David B. Chamberlain, Ph.D.

Author, *The Mind of Your Newborn Baby* (North Atlantic Books, 1998)

Editor, *Birthpsychology.com*

# Introduction

In the autumn of 1977, I flew to Seoul, Korea with only a child's violin in hand and one hundred dollars in my pocket. I'd come to meet someone with whom I'd exchanged one hundred and one "love letters," but whom I'd seen only through a single photograph — smiling, in her late twenties, dark braids, a puffy pink and white dress, posing behind long pink and white cosmos flowers. Was she fat, or thin? She even could have been pregnant, but, of course, she wasn't!

Young Im *(Root of Responsibility)* greeted me at Kimpo Airport with a great, shy smile and then whisked me off in a taxi to a small, secluded room in the hills. Three months later, we were wed, adorned like a traditional king and queen, in a Buddhist temple on a snowy mountaintop.

My romance with the folk customs of Korea, as well as those of neighboring China and Japan grew, especially when, four years later, it came time for us to bear a child. My wife then introduced me to the child-bearing tradition of the twelfth century B.C., Queen Jin, or Ta Jen of Chou (a small kingdom in China), one which would influence our own children's destinies.

Queen Ta Jen (太任), whose name in Chinese characters means, "Great Responsibility," is called, "The Great Mother of the Unborn Child," for her practice of the art of *T'ai Chiao* (胎教) while her son, the future sage-king Wen and author of the classic *I-Ching* ("The Book of Changes") was in her womb. The Chinese character *T'ai* (胎) represents variously, "Womb, Embryo, Fetus, Umbilical Cord, or Placenta." *Chiao* (教) is "Education ('to nourish or cause to grow')". Together, the ideograms mean "Embryonic Education." Queen Jin's manner of *T'ai Chiao* was adopted by royal and aristocratic women, their servants, and other commoners throughout China,

1

then outside of the country, primarily in Korea, where it is pronounced *T'ae Gyo*, and in Japan, *Tai Kyu*.

Kim Jo Shin, a Confucian sage in Korea, explains the essence of *Embryonic Education*. "Almost all women think the fetus in the womb is not yet a human being. So they spend ten months of very valuable time in quite an empty way. They don't think seriously about their responsibilities.

In the old days, people saw the necessity for *T'ae Gyo* and so gave a pure education, in a variety of ways, to the fetus.

Before beginning, you should assume that the fetus in your womb is a normal person, who deserves to be treated like a human being (for this reason, I have sparingly used the impersonal term "it" to refer to the baby, preferring "he," "she," or "(s)he" in random sections).

The method of education involves giving the baby endless love and communication through the vibration of minds. If a father and mother have a deep love for each other, are faithful to each other, and devote themselves wholly to their baby, it will grow normally."

A child is "pure" upon conception and more receptive to any "good" or "bad" influences during pregnancy than it will ever be after it is born. What could be better than those of loving, cooperative parents? From them one learns how to be a full-hearted human being.

In Korea, because of the age-old belief in a thriving and receptive life in the womb, from conception on, a baby is already reckoned as one-year old at birth. This is why a sensitive mother, recognizing the importance of *Embryonic Education*, single-mindedly aims to create a living work of art in her womb.

At the Lotus Lantern Buddhist Center in Seoul, during a dream workshop I was facilitating, Gabriella, her blue eyes sparkling with joy, told me her dream of years ago in Italy:

A little boy took a train into the countryside. It passed through what was called on a sign, "The Tunnel of Life and Death," into a deep forest. Then it curled around a tall mountain to the top. There, the little boy got off the train and met an old man. He was a teacher of sculpture. He had the clay model of a human before him and said,

"I am trying to make the perfect human." The little boy, in imitation, picked up a pile of fallen leaves, mashing them all together, but they just crumbled to dust. He shrugged his shoulders helplessly. The old man smiled, for it wasn't so easy to make a perfect human.

He said, "Look out on the world there." They peered over a cliff; down below was the world and so many people in the towns and cities. "See what a hard life they have. We must do something to help them."

When I heard Gabriella's dream, I felt that it concerned being re-formed, sculpting her own inner self into that of a perfect human, capable of enriching the lives of others. I suggested that she recall the potentials of this dream whenever feeling down.

Similarly, can a pregnant woman and her spouse take advantage of the opportunity to affect the quality of their baby, and also to reshape their own lives, by developing into more sensitive, cooperative human beings and, consequentially, contributing to a more caring society?

I am grateful for the help of the following people, who have generously helped give birth to this guide: my wife and daughters; students and colleagues at Hankuk University of Foreign Studies; Oriental Medical Doctors at Kyunghee University and other friends in Seoul, South Korea; Dr. David Chamberlain of APPPAH; Richard Grossinger, Lindy Hough, Chris Pitts, Jennifer Dunn, Jennifer Privateer, and the rest of the staff at North Atlantic Books, as well as many others.

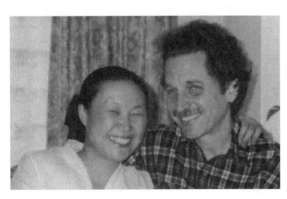

Fred J. Seligson
Seoul, South Korea

*Young Im and Fred Jeremy Seligson*

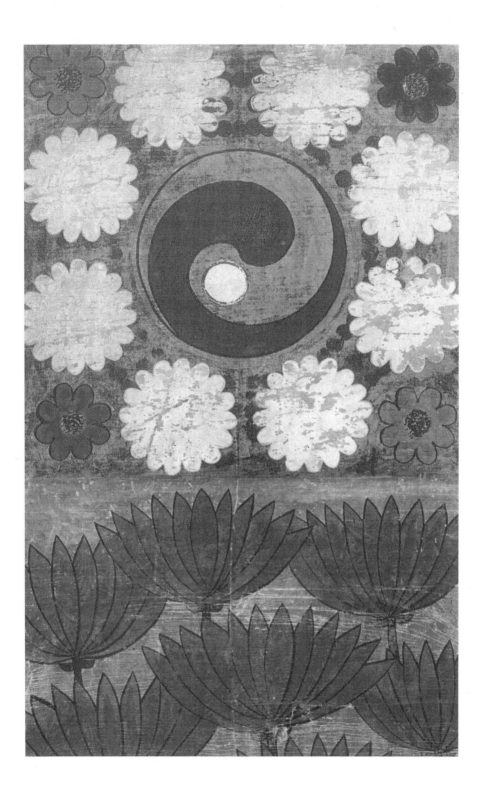

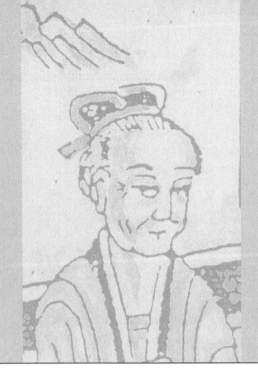

# Preparing for Conception

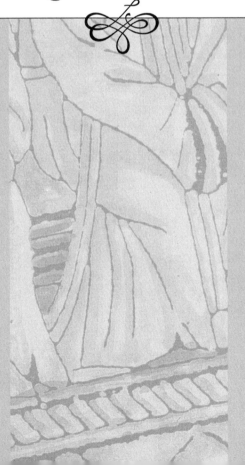

*The first birth of our people*
*Was from Chiang Yuan.*

*How did she give birth to (our) people?*
*That her childlessness be taken away.*

*She then trod on a toe-print made by God,*
*And was moved,*
*In the large place where she rested.*

*She became pregnant; she dwelt retired;*
*She gave birth to and nourished (a son),*
*Who was Hou Chi.*

*When she had fulfilled her months,*
*Her first-born (came forth) like a lamb.*

*There was no bursting or rending,*
*No injury, no hurt,*
*Showing how wonderful he could be.*

*Did God not give her comfort?*
*Had he not accepted her pure offering and sacrifice,*
*So that thus easily she brought forth her son?*

—*The Book of Odes* (1,000 B.C.) [2]


*       *       *


*A child's education begins one hundred days before*
*conception.*

—Korean Saying

*All*
*beauty*

*comes*
*from*
*beautiful*
*thoughts*

*through*
*our*
*lives.*

*Beauty*
*at*
*birth*

*comes*
*from*
*beauty*

*in*
*the*
*womb;*

*beauty*
*in*
*the*
*womb*

*comes*
*from*
*beautiful*
*thoughts*

*&*

*before*
*that,*

*beautifully*
*thought*
*ovum*
*&*
*sperm.*

*Beauty*
*at*
*conception*

*comes*
*from*
*beautiful*
*thoughts,*

*mother's*
*father's*
*grandmother's*
*grandfather's,*

*all the family*
*on back*
*to Adam*
*(or Africa).*

*When*
*beautiful*
*thoughts*
*end*

*our*
*wrongs*
*begin.*

—F. J. S.

# Praying for a Baby

Yun Hui wakes up before sunrise, bathes, dons clean white clothes, then climbs up a hill to a shrine. There, she prays for a son to carry on the family name. Only if she already has a son, might she pray for the companionship of a daughter.

She believes that if she offers sacrifices of rice, water, and wine and prays with sincerity, her words can reach the ears of the local mountain god, or else those of the Seven Stars God, who has the power to direct a baby spirit to her womb.

During one hundred days of purification and prayer, she proves herself worthy of conceiving a child and also prepares to be a caring mother.

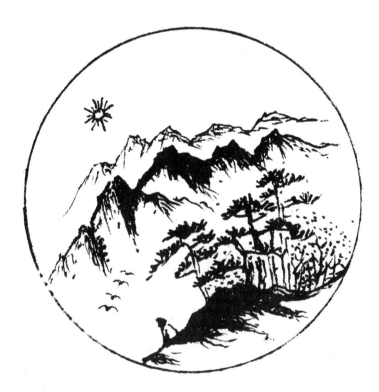

*May a lovely child come into my womb.*

8

## Moon Child

What a mother-to-be thinks of or acts on during the day tends to appear symbolically in her dreams: "In my mother's dream," relates Miss Hong, a university student,

> *it was night, but the moon's light made it as bright as day. The wind became quiet. Only an owl's cry broke the silence. Mother stepped out in the yard, wearing a (billowy) Korean dress. An old, branchy tree was there. She scooped a bowl of clean water out of a well, took it under the tree, and started praying for a child. She prayed very earnestly. Then rays of moonlight came down on her wide skirt in a shining line. She was greatly surprised and instinctively hugged them in her arms.*

"It is said that it will be a daughter if moonbeams come down to a mother, and a son if rays of sunlight do. So I, a girl, was conceived after this dream."

## Mother of a Holy Child

*Anxious, my heart fluttering, I opened the back door and looked up into the night. The hills were all silver behind our cottage; the trees were silver bows, the shrubs silver arrows, and the grass silver spears. Those silver breasts of graves I wanted to suck, and the moon was almost at the full of silvery brightness, so bright I could not look directly at it.*

*I shielded my eyes and effortlessly crawled through the grasses and wet flowers to the top of the highest mound, my grandfather's. So high and round, so smooth and deliciously wet, it seemed to reach up to the moon.*

*As I lay there in the fresh grasses, all silvery myself, I felt I could touch the moon, lay my hand on it, and I stretched out my slender arm and felt with my fingers its delicate surface. The moon was misty, silvery. It was shining and pleasant to see. My hands were silver, soft and white crimson; my fingers melted and all I could see was you.*

9

*You, my dear! Instead of a moon, there was an empty place, filled with a million colors. A perfect diaphanous sphere, an ocean splashing in a globe, and inside a baby, floating in the sea, with kindly, though mischievous eyes, gazing at me. Ah, from an incredible void, from the heavens, a child. Ah, this is life in its wonderful magnitude. Ah, I never knew this could be.*

*"Come to me, little one, little boy!" I cried, for it was one, I could plainly see. He was naked, too, save for the halo of the moon around his head and the rainbow of the sun encircling his body. His dark pearly eyes were piercing as if they could see through to the center of my deepest secrets, laying all bare. And he spoke, the baby spoke to me, "Dear woman, fear not for me to see you as you are; that is how all should see one another. All melts into the dew and merges with silver rays, rising each morning off the sweet grasses back into the sun, our father. A cloud is all we are, formed by the moon and melted by the sun. Open wide your womb, open up your home. It is time for me to come inside."*

## Prayers to the Dragon King

My wife, Young Im, shares a story:

My father's mother had been unable to conceive during several years of marriage. In despair, she and her husband finally adopted her brother-in-law's second son, so that they could have an heir to their vast family estate, which included a lovely pavilion overlooking the scenic Kum Gang River near Puyo (South Korea). Grandmother, however, still wanted to bear a son of her own, so every fifteen days, on the full and new moons, she would climb down to the winding riverbank to bathe, make an offering of rice and wine, and pray to the Dragon King for a son. The Dragon King, who dwells in all bodies of water, is the god of procreation.

Grandmother would also offer a gift of seaweed and rice to her servant women whenever one gave birth to a baby. By so blessing the children of others, she believed that she was acquiring merit to deserve her own in the eyes of the Dragon King. One night, she dreamt of seeing a very powerful dragon and woke up elated. The women's quarters were separate from the men's. In Confucian society, the man always visits his wife in her quarters, for it is considered unmannerly if the woman goes to her husband's room for lovemaking. Grandmother, however, was so impressed by the dream that she hurried over to his room and seduced him. Her audacity is why she was nicknamed, 'Tiger Lady.' Soon she was pregnant with a son.

Even so, out of fear of offending their relative's family, they kept their adopted son as the sole heir. Grandmother's husband died early, leaving her a young widow. Her only wish was for her sons to 'fill the house with grandchildren.' Their adopted son fathered nine children, and her natural son fathered twelve, one of whom is my mother.

## A Prayer

When a woman reaches her place of prayer (even if a clean alcove in her own house), she surrounds herself with an invisible shawl of stillness. She sits or stands silently with hands comfortably folded together for a few minutes, allowing tranquility to flow through. She lets a cool, clean breeze come blow freshness into her body and soul, leaving all troubles behind. She asks the object of her faith:

> *"Respectable Spirit (or "Holy Mother/Father") please cleanse my body and soul so I might receive a good, healthy baby."*

## Lovemaking by the Stars

Two hundred and fifty years ago, a father stationed on the Chinese frontier sent a letter home:

Dear Son,

Your mother wrote that you are getting married; I'm glad to hear it. Now, there are several suggestions that I'd like to make to you. You ought to follow them in order to produce a good, healthy child, one who's easy to rear....

Once you and your spouse have been living compatibly and are prepared to bring up a child in an atmosphere of joy, consult a doctor or a qualified astrologer, who can select auspicious *egg days* for making love. By choosing carefully, you can increase the chances of conceiving a healthy, star-blessed child.

Select your *egg days* so as to enjoy a fair weather season, ten (lunar) months later, for giving birth to your baby. Spring is fitting because nature is becoming manifest: wild greens and flowers are erupting, bird eggs are hatching and other baby creatures are appearing on farms and in nearby forests. Spring is mild, so the mother can care for an infant more safely then. Autumn can be as congenial, a time of harvest, plenty.

Make sure that the days for lovemaking are mild and clear. The air should be fresh, carrying the chirping of birds and at night twinkling with stars and perhaps fireflies. Such an atmosphere is soothing to you and your future child.

But, if it is windy, rainy, with booming thunder and flashing lightning, or if the sun or moon is in eclipse, these are not good occasions for making love. Such disturbances could cut your baby's life short and affect his brain.

Choose a clean, respectable residence where you won't be disturbed. Let a few hours lapse after dining.

Before entering the nuptial chamber, bathe. By no means get drunk, because you could lose sight of your sacred purpose—a loving child—and sow the seeds for a lustful one. You and your wife's feelings will be carried over to your son or daughter at the moment of conception.

During lovemaking, you need only arouse moderate desire; strong passions tend to scatter the emanations. Rather than lusting, it is better for you and your spouse to perceive yourselves as co-creators of a lovely child.

If, after several months, you have trouble conceiving, climb up a secluded hill and expose yourself to the vitalizing rays of the early morning sun, but make sure nobody's aunt is picking herbs up there!

As for your wife, she might sip the condensed *ch'i* (bio-energy) of dew from grasses at dawn, dance with other young women in spirals under the full moon, or else drink the moon reflected in a bowl of water.

During lovemaking, wait for your wife to get excited first, so that the old blood from her womb is discharged before you ejaculate. This way, new blood can be generated and the vagina can open its two small ducts, the right for female essence and the left for male essence. You give and she receives. All results in something beautiful, like the making of gold through alchemy.

Ask her to be open to your embrace. Retaining the presence of mind to ask her how she is feeling is helpful for consummation. Appreciating each other's offer of, and need for, affection furthers unity of purpose.

Also, it could help to pray for the child's welfare—while making love.

A son is favored in our country, because he is the heir to the family name and estate, supporter of his parents in old age, and keeper of ancestral rites. Daughters, no matter how much adored, are normally lost to other families after marriage.

I know of several instances of frustrated couples, like the Chows, who persisted in making a string of daughters until finally after four, five, or more they finally bore a son and, then, relieved, haha, refrained from producing any other children.

Still, once a son is born, the joy of a frolicsome little girl in the house is often sought after and appreciated, especially by a hen-pecked father; oh how well I know this! If he cares for her, she will reward him with undying affection and be a delightful companion, but if he ignores her, she, in return, could shun him and conceive a prejudice against men.

As for your wife, a daughter can be of great value in helping around the house: cooking, cleaning, or bringing up younger siblings; moreover, she can be cheerful company as long as she is treated kindly.

Waiting for the good news,

Your Father [3]

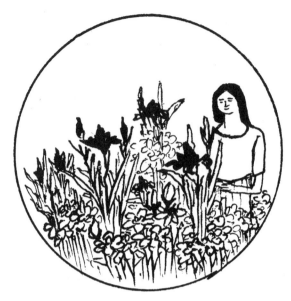

*Before carrying a flower of my own,*
*I'll grow a beautiful one in my mind.*

## Dreaming of Conception

*A white snake*
*follows her,*
*but strangely,*
*she's unafraid;*
*it's pretty*
*and loveable.*
*She walks*
*the rest of the way*
*while playing*
*with the snake.*

I was conceived after this dream.

\*　　\*　　\*

Growing up in a small village, Yun Hui overhears her mother and other women discuss babies at the well or by the stream. She gath-

14

ers that conception is a reward for prayers and sacrifices to the Seven Stars God, or a family ancestor, called the Three Gods Grandmother, who carries the baby spirit to the womb and later guards it on through birth. Conception is announced by a dream, called a *T'ae Mong* (胎夢) or "Fetus Dream" which every mother-to-be has. A *T'ae Mong* is sent from the other world, and is a highly coveted message.

Yun Hui learns how to determine the sex, character, health, and destiny of a newly-conceived child through a *T'ae Mong;* this knowledge becomes an intuitive part of her being as she grows up. Within her is a dream-divination system, founded on local folk beliefs, as well as Taoist categories of feminine and masculine or *yin/yang* qualities. As were those of generations of mothers and fathers before her, her heart-mind,[4] when the time comes, will become a net for catching her own conception dream.

She comes of age, and her marriage is arranged by a matchmaker to a stranger from a distant village. An auspicious date for the wedding is also chosen and the solemn, often tearful event is held. She is only sixteen years old. Romantic love has never been a factor; that is something which is expected to grow naturally as the life-long bond progresses.

Several months pass, then her mother-in-law starts badgering her to produce a son. Yun Hui ties blue threads around her big toes to attract a boy's spirit. The couple visits a fortuneteller, who divines auspicious days for intercourse, which they must memorize and religiously observe. On chosen dates, the father-in-law sends his son into the nuptial chamber with the admonition, "Make a son!"

After this fails, Yun Hui makes offerings of rice and pure water, while devotedly praying for one hundred days to the local mountain god before a phallus-shaped stone on a cliff, but nothing comes of this.

One afternoon, exhausted by her day's labors, she curls up on a straw mat for a nap, and dreams:

*She crosses a dirt road, on the verge of a woods, then suddenly a huge, black bear appears before her. Scared, she runs straight for her house. But when she flings open the doors, she finds that the bear is already sitting comfortably on the floor inside.*

This astonishing spectacle wakes her. She sits up, heart skipping a beat and racing on. Catching her breath, she hurries over to her mother-in-law, in the kitchen, and blurts out, "I've just had an awful dream!"

Having listened to the passionate account, her mother-in-law gives a sigh of relief and just smiles. A few days later, in a dream:

> *Yun Hui encounters the bear again. Before she can run away, it suddenly lunges and bites her hand.*

Waking up, she exclaims, "Ah…!," for she recognizes that she is pregnant, *and* with the spirit of a bear-like child. She also divines that it will be a boy, because she has heard that a large, aggressive animal in a dream signifies one.

After their initial excitement over these "Fetus Dreams," her mother-in-law admonishes her, "Don't tell anybody else, because a dream has a special power of its own. Each time it is told, its charm diminishes."

Mother-in-law even advises her, "Don't tell your child before he is thirty years old," to ensure the magical power of the dream and his own success in life.

Yun Hui turns the dreams over in her thoughts during pregnancy, imprinting the characteristics of a bear on the delicate fetal heart. If the child were not already endowed with the traits of a bear, he would be encouraged to acquire some by the emotionally-colored images he receives through the communion of his mother's heart and his own.

## "Moon Essence"

Young Im narrates, "My mother bore my elder sister in 1946, then a few years later, my brother, but he died one hundred days after birth. Next, I was born, then two more daughters. So she started to worry about the absence of a male heir.

"My father said, 'Don't fret, it doesn't matter if we have sons or daughters. Nonetheless, the next time my mother was pregnant, I followed her to a nearby Chinese Medicine shop, where she was going to buy herbs. I remember the doctor. He was a gentle old man with a clear face and a long, white beard, like a Taoist. The name of the shop was 'Moon Essence.' Mother drank his medicine and ten months later, my brother, Chul Ho, was born."

## Ingredients of the Moon

In 1992, during one of my calls to his office, Dr. Choi Seung Hoon, O.M.D., who teaches Oriental Pathology at Kyunghee University in Seoul, unveiled to me his own secret formula for encouraging fertility and, in particular, a son. It worked in the instance of his second child, a much-coveted boy. His way has three requirements: 1) the drinking of a certain mixture of herbal medicine 2) a specific period for imbibing the herbs, and 3) the manner of making love.

Dr. Choi's special formula serves to stimulate the *ch'i*, or the life force, in the stagnated blood and the mother's reproductive organs, to create an environment conducive to conceiving a son.

The seven dried herbs include a rhizome, *Attractylodes macrocephala koidz* (12 grams); a fungus, *Poria* (8 grams); White peony root (8 grams); *Rehmannia Root* (8 grams); Chinese Yam (8 grams); Dogwood Fruit (6 grams); and Safflower (2 grams). They are mixed together in a pack and boiled at the woman's home in a clay pot over a low flame for an hour to an hour and a half. Or, for the convenience of these busy days, an herbalist can boil them in his office and seal them in plastic bags for single doses taken an hour before meals.

This brew should be consumed by the woman three times a day, for ten days, from the beginning of her menstrual cycle. Then, between the seventh and twenty-first days of the cycle, when conception is possible, the couple should make love. Also, if the total of the couple's ages results in an even number, the lunar months for making love must be odd-numbered ones, like January, March, May, etc. If the sum is an odd number, then the months should be even ones, such as February, April, June, and so forth.

As for the manner of making love, "When the woman gets

excited first, an alkaline environment is created by her fluids in her vagina, and this is suitable for conducting a male sperm. However, if the man is excited first, then an acidic environment remains, favoring the female sperm."

In 1993, I visited Dr. Hwang Dae Suk, a white-bearded, eighty-one-year-old folk practitioner in the Korean countryside, who claims, "Out of 3,000 cases, I have failed only seven times to produce a pregnancy with my herbs." His clinic is so packed that he sets a limit of sixty persons a day. My wife, daughter, and I had to sleep outside his office door overnight just to reserve a place for him to check our pulses.

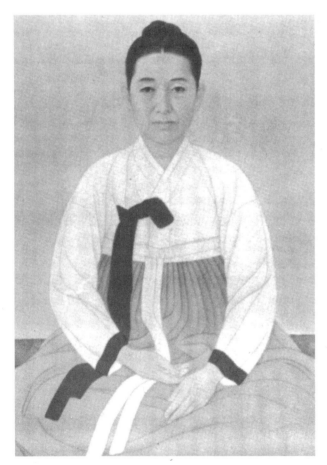

*Lady Sim Sa Im Dang, "Teacher of Responsibility"; gifted poetess and painter, mother of the great neo-Confucian philosopher Lee Yul Guk. (Portrait by Kim Un Ho, 1955. Courtesy of Kangnung O Juk'un Municipal Museum, Korea.)*

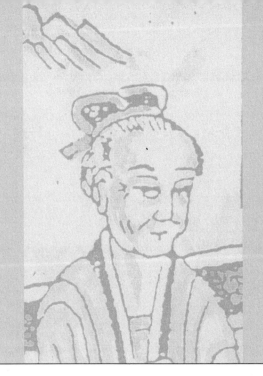

# Cultivating Your Flower

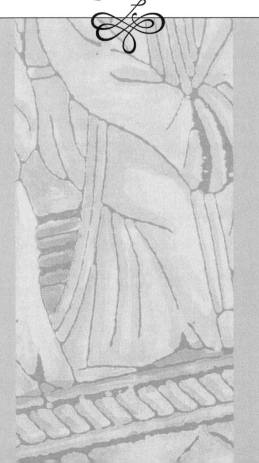

*The hand belongs to the regions of the lesser Yin. When the motion of the pulse is great, she is with child.*

—*The Yellow Emperor's Classic of Internal Medicine* [5]

*       *       *

*All creatures depend on Embryonic Education, even insects!*

—Lee Jae Young, eighty-four-year-old Korean folk doctor

*       *       *

*When a phoenix hatches a sweet-hearted chick, we can appreciate the value of a mother's tenderness and fairness to her baby.*

*On the other hand, as soon as a tiger cub or a wolf pup is born, it already has a greedy and violent disposition. This is due to the cruel ways its mother behaved while she was pregnant.*

*We must recall such examples when raising our own children. A tigress's cub has not received good teaching in the womb. So it is prone to harm other animals and people, too.*

*This is a lesson of Embryonic Education.*

—Ja Hee, *The New Record* (130 B.C.)

*Jin, the second of the princesses of Chu
from (the domain of) Yin Shang,*

*came to be married to the prince of Chou, and
became his wife in the capital.*

*Both she and King Chi were entirely virtuous;
(then) Ta Jen became pregnant, and gave birth*

*to our own King Wen.*

—The Book of Odes [6]

\*   \*   \*

*The superior man will say that Ta Jen could commence
the instruction of her child while he was yet in the womb.*

—Lu Hiang's commentary on *The Book of Odes* [7]

# Queen Jin's Rules

Queen Jin, or Ta Jen *(Great Responsibility)* is revered in China, Taiwan, Korea, and Japan for her behavior while pregnant with the sage-king Wen (author of the classic *I-Ching*) in the twelfth century B.C. She also guided her daughter-in-law, Queen Ssu, in her pregnancy with the sage-king Wu (who expanded on his father's work). Lu Hiang, in his *A Loyal and Virtuous Woman's Story* (first century A.D.) enlightens us:

"Every night before retiring, Ta Jen would ask a blind musician to sing her songs about great men of the past. By listening to these, she hoped to bear a child of upright character and talent. Also, before the queen fell asleep, the blind man would be requested to remind her of the correct things a pregnant woman should do in order to safely bear a good, healthy child. He would reply respectfully to the highly regarded lady, whose character we are told was firm and constant:

> To avoid a miscarriage, don't lay on your side, or sit with one leg folded under you, or squat on a rough surface. Generally, if a place doesn't feel right for you, don't sit there.
>
> Regarding food for the baby, if it doesn't taste good, don't eat anymore. And, if it isn't cut neatly—square, round or evenly—don't eat it.
>
> Considering your baby's feelings, don't look at dirty or gloomy colors. Don't listen to lewd sounds, like a debaucher's voice. Don't speak arrogantly, or ill of others.

Finally, the blind man would remind her,

> When you go to sleep, lay your body in a comfortable, plain position."

Then he would leave her alone to contemplate and, perhaps, dream of his words. When she awoke the next morning, the rules for her appropriate behavior would seem second nature, and she would be able to follow them effortlessly.

Lu concludes the queen's biography, "An expectant mother must be able to exercise self-control, so as to sustain good feelings and avoid encouraging the bad, if she wishes to produce a good child, one with the wisdom and virtue of the noble sons of Queens Ta Jen and Ta Ssu of the Chou dynasty. Otherwise, if ill feelings exist, a bad-mannered child will be born."

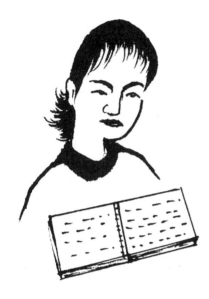

*I'll follow the rules of* Embryonic Education *and become a good mother.*

## Yun Hui: a Korean Bride

Yun Hui and others have been squatting and scrubbing, drumming their soaped-up family garments with sticks on flat rocks, chattering away. The path up the bank is slippery, but Yun Hui's household clothes have to be spotlessly clean.

Underneath the basket of clothes, her long, plaited hair is wet and cool, for she had washed it, as well, by the stream. It is rolled about in loops, balancing the load.

A dirt road twists here and there around shady oaks and enormous stones. Yun Hui weaves against a strong breeze that is fingering its way between gnarled pines. And feeling chilly, she picks her way nimbly around potholes.

Soon smokestacks, poking out of the clay sides of thatched dwellings, appear. A yellow dog runs out barking, only to turn lazily back. Yun Hui pushes open the rickety gate to a small, dirt yard, where a few long, pink and white cosmos flowers have managed to bloom, and steps over to a line strung between two trees. She set her burden down and starts hanging the clothes up to dry in the breeze.

Her grandmother-in-law, a gray-haired woman with a shrunken-apple face, calls raspingly to her from the porch, "Yun Hui, I would advise you to take it easy and to follow as many of these customary, Seven Rules for *Embryonic Education* as you can:

*First*, for the baby's safety:
Don't wash your long hair during the month before giving birth; you could catch cold outdoors.

Don't sit on a backless chair, climb on a ledge, up a rock or a steep hill, cross rugged paths or raging streams, or carry loads.

Also, abstain from drinking wine and eating unusual foods.

*Second:*
Don't chatter away with your friends to no good purpose, or let yourself be surprised by anything.

Also, keep from laughing hysterically over a joke, or crying out for someone's attention.

These are ways to waste energy, harm the character of, and even miscarry, your baby.

*Third:*
Avoid sitting on other people's chairs (could fall off) during the first month of pregnancy. Take care around windows and doors (could get a surprise) in the second; thresholds, in the third; fireplaces, in the fourth ; wooden beds, in the fifth; stairwells, in the sixth ; rooms by a gate, in the seventh; the water closet (could give birth prematurely) in the eighth; and stationery shops (so the baby doesn't get an early congratulatory note!) in the ninth.

*Fourth*:
Sit quietly, listening to beautiful words; sing and play your harp. Memorize poems and the precepts of sages. In this manner, your

baby can become peaceful, artistic, and wise.

So as to guard the baby's disposition against evil influences, don't listen to foul-mouthed speech or look upon unpleasant scenes or conceive ill feelings toward others.

*Fifth:*

Lest you slip and injure your baby, don't balance your weight on one foot only, lay your body across any object, or lean against anything for support.

*Sixth*:

To refine your baby's character, hold a piece of white jade in your palm or dangle a jade pendant over your belly.

Wear a soothing perfume.

Hang a painting of a Chinese phoenix or of a sea turtle, each of whom is a praiseworthy mother to its young, beside your bed. Say aloud, "I'm going to be a mother just like you!"

*Seventh:*

To avoid injuring your baby or creating a lusty atmosphere that might stain his (or her) character, live a chaste life, without sexual intercourse. Don't worry, I'll talk to my grandson about it, too.

Of course, there's no need for me to say this, but if you commit adultery during the month of parturition, your baby could become ill or even die. He could be shocked by the act, as well as poisoned by his mother's disloyalty and shame.

If you observe these teachings faithfully, you'll have no trouble giving birth to a good-looking, healthy child; one with a bright and sensitive mind, emulating your own.

"By the way, Yun Hui, you looked back at me over your left shoulder when I called your name; this means you're probably bearing a son!"

Yun Hui says, "Do I have to follow all those rules? It's so difficult for me."

The old woman frowns and replies, "If so, there is a way I heard from my own grandmother-in-law. The main idea is that you and the child are continually connected body and heart. You are no longer one person, but two. So, you must live your days in a sincere way to benefit your child.

25

"Sit quietly under those old pines, inhale the fresh air, and listen to the sound of a breeze blowing through the needles. It can give you and your child a deep, understanding heart."

*"I'll try my best."*

## Mrs. Lee's "New Theory"

Mrs. Lee Sa Ju Dang authored the celebrated *New Theory of Embryonic Education (T'ae Gyo Shingi)* (1801). By writing in the vernacular Korean alphabet *(Han Gul)* rather than in the usual Chinese characters, which could be understood only by the aristocratic, ruling class, she could reach out for a wide, female audience. She died before publication, but the book was popularized by her son Yu Gyeong, a noted scholar of the Korean alphabet and a fine product of education in her womb. Two hundred years later, Sa Ju Dang's teachings are still being observed by Koreans. She counseled:

When pregnant, a woman ought to avoid (among others):
- Overdressing, or making her body too hot or cold.
- Overeating.
- Oversleeping.
- Sitting somewhere too hot or too cold, in a dirty place, or on an edge.
- Climbing to a high place.
- Going out at night.
- Joining an excursion to the fields or mountains.
- Glancing down a well, or at an old grave.
- Entering a funeral house.
- Passing along a sheer mountain road.
- Carrying a heavy burden.
- Placing all her weight on her left (less steady) foot, leaning against a pillar.
- Going into a dangerous place or hurrying.
- Getting acupuncture or cauterized with *moxa* (dry mugwort) in a careless fashion, or taking medicines indiscriminately....

She should straighten her body when climbing up and lean forward when climbing down.

According to a doctor, if a woman who is pregnant catches a chill or a cold, her baby will, too. If she gets a fever, so will her baby.

If she grasps this, she will understand why getting soaked or parched or slumping halfway over or all the way down is not good for a pumpkin. In the same way a pumpkin is affected by the condition of its roots, a baby is by his mother's condition.

If she is not careful with her health, how can she gather the strength to educate her child? If she fails to do so fully, she won't be able to bring up a baby of natural talents and long life.

She should always try to be happy, maintain a peaceful mind and pure heart, be generous to others, mild and genial, without carrying it (falsely) to an extreme."

Sa Ju Dang, whose chosen name means *Teacher of the Unborn Child* contributed to the cultivation of feminine virtues and to the development of good-mannered children, ones who could grow up to contribute to their society. She believed that a child is "pure" at conception, and that it was a mother's duty to keep it that way through her examples of careful, healthy living. Therefore, she wrote:

Education in the womb is a mother's responsibility. It is not just a courtesy to the child. Being conceived from one's father, educated by one's mother and taught by a teacher are all interconnected. Ten (lunar) months of education during pregnancy are of more importance than ten years of learning from a teacher after birth.

The Confucian goal of training a child in the womb, according to Sa Ju Dang, was to "teach a child to be a true gentleman, so he will do the right things, even for generations. If he doesn't become a gentleman, his mother should be scolded, because a fetus is influenced by its mother's behavior, by what she eats, drinks, sees, hears, thinks, and feels. She must not see, hear, speak, do, or even think evil."

A proverb adds, "A woman's body is not just her own. The baby in her womb is also a member of the family."

27

Sa Ju Dang writes, "A man who does not attend to his child's needs in the womb is equal to an animal."

On the other hand, a folk expression goes, "If a man can care for his wife's emotional needs, then he has the ability to be a good father to their child."

Also, "A father's care for his wife during pregnancy is more important than that of ten other relatives."

One's spouse should follow a decent daily routine, one filled with compassion for others. If he comes home in a good, relaxed mood (perhaps after exercise, or meditation), he can cater to the needs of his wife, speak softly, and contribute to her happiness.

*A page written in* Hangul, *(Korean alphabet) from the original* New Theory of Embryonic Education *by Lady Lee Sa Ju Dang, "Mother of the Unborn Child"*

# Soothing Morning Sickness

Yun Hui is advised by her mother-in-law to stay busy during pregnancy. "Doing light chores can relieve morning sickness."

Leisurely, she dusts and sweeps the house. She wanders about ventilating rooms with fresh air and sunlight, sprinkling water on plants, and so forth. While putting her own house in order, she is also doing the same for the baby's.

## Figure 8

When my wife, Young Im, suffered from morning sickness during her pregnancy, she found relief in the Figure 8 exercise created by Neeshi Katsuo (1894–1959), a Japanese health authority.

With arms and legs raised off the ground, she would amble on all fours, like a little bear, in a Figure 8, on our living-room floor. After some minutes, she usually felt relieved.

She says, "Neeshi observed that four-legged animals rarely experienced morning sickness. Since ages ago we too ambled on all fours and carried our young suspended underneath, when a pregnant woman tries to walk in this way, it reduces nausea and dizziness. Why a Figure 8? It's less boring than a circle."

After ambling about, she would rest for a few minutes.

Young Im practiced another exercise called Cells Dancing as part of Neeshi's program.

She would lie on her back, neck supported on a low, curved, wooden pillow, and lift her arms and legs at a ninety degree angle. Then she would start shaking loosely from the ends of her fingers and toes in a slow, steady rhythm for three to five minutes, followed by a minute or two of rest. The sensation is similar to what one feels in an idling bus. "Cells Dancing" stimulates all the body's cells.

Still supine, Young Im would continue with "Uniting Hands and Feet," setting her soles together, and her palms, too, as if praying. The upper digits of her middle fingers would be touching firmly.

Like rowing a boat, she would slowly, rhythmically extend her fingers and toes in opposite directions along the carpet and then draw them back again, raising her hands beyond her head, for a few minutes at a time. Then she would close up, hands above the heart, and rest quietly.

She says, "It felt so cool and relaxing. After I began labor, about 9 P.M., the contractions were very small, but, later, I couldn't sleep because of the pain coming about every ten minutes. So, I did this exercise slowly, and it relieved the pain. Toward the end, when the pain was worse, lying quietly with my palms together was especially comforting.

"Also, you got me laughing a lot by making fun of me. That's why our first daughter laughs a lot now!"

This pair of exercises aided Young Im's circulation, kept her body limber, and contributed to her fairly easy labor and delivery (as well as, I guess, to the subsequent tireless activity and amazing strength of our slender girl's legs. My mother-in-law exclaimed, "That baby looks like she's riding a bicycle!"). I recall Young Im's exercising at about 4 A.M. on the sofa, just before she sent me out for a taxi to carry her to the hospital for delivery.

She suggests: "A smaller baby will be borne by a woman who does a lot of exercise. This contributes to an easier birth. Don't worry, the baby can be fattened up afterwards."

## Sleeping with Child

Young Im says, "A pillow stuffed with wild chrysanthemums is cooling for the brain. It was a favorite of dandy Korean scholars."

The proverbial "cool head and warm feet" could also assist pregnant mothers.

Japanese professor Kyoshi Oshima, Ph.D., of Kyoto University, in his guide, *T'ae Kyu* (1988), counsels a woman carrying a baby to "first lie down on your side, then roll over slowly without jarring your body. If you lean straight back, you could startle your baby, impeding his free movements. Then, he is apt to kick his feet excitedly."

Shift about until you feel comfortable, as long as you don't lie with your belly on a pillow. You may rest on a side, but keep your spine straight. The right (liver) side will cool your body off and the left (heart) side will heat it up.

"Sleep in a quiet, well-darkened bedroom," continues Professor Oshima. "Follow a regular pattern of retiring early, depending on the season; for example, in spring, around 8 or 9 P.M., and waking early about 6 A.M., with the rising sun. This is reassuring to the baby, who grows accustomed to his mother's routine. However, if it is irregular, he is apt to be nervous after birth."

## Three Lovers

Chinese sages observed that animals in a state of nature abstained from intercourse while pregnant, so it was considered unnatural for humans to make love then. Yet, it's true, sometimes a baby's heart does beat rapidly in the womb, partly in response to her parents, and even out of fear, when they are passionately making love.

According to a Western-trained physician, Kim Chang Kyu, M.D., professor of Obstetrics and Gynecology at Yonsei University in Seoul, who appeared on MBC T.V., March 6, 2000, if a woman has a propensity to miscarry, then it is not prudent for her to make love at all during pregnancy. For others, during the first few months, because the baby might not be secure in the womb, it is also advisable to forego making love then.

For those who are disappointed by this news, take heart, for Dr. Kim also says that a safe period is normally from the sixteenth to the twentieth week, when the baby's body and limbs have assumed full-term proportions, and it is securely floating in the womb. During that month, if a couple makes love adoringly, the baby could respond with joyful movements, opening her lips and sucking on her fingers, or playing with the umbilical cord. Later on, the wall of the womb progressively thins, and the baby grows closer to the surface.

Dr. Kim suggests that the parents' attitude toward, and, manner of, enjoyment of sex is transferred from the parents heart on down to the child and becomes part of her *Embryonic Education.*

## For Healthy Bones

*Close your eyes. Sit relaxed, breathing rhythmically from the pelvis.*

*Join all of your bones, by way of thought, gradually to the warm South, to Tibet, and the planet Pluto.*

*Feel your bones growing warm, elastic, and stronger.*

## Dining with a Guest

Cool, fresh water is essential for a mother and child; whatever Mother consumes, so does Baby.

Choi Seung Hoon, O.M.D., declares in his office at Kyunghee University in Seoul, "Piping hot drinks raise a mother's already high body temperature and increase the fetal heart rate, but icy drinks lower her temperature and decrease the fetal heart rate. A habit of ice-cold drinks can harm her hard-working kidneys (and consequently, bones)."

### Tea and Juice

"Plain green tea is too cold in nature for a baby," cautions Jang Gi Nam, O.M.D., who treats patients at the Shin Nong Baek Cho clinic, "but brown rice-green tea is a perfect combination."

Kyunghee's Pak Chon Guk, O.M.D., says, "Osage orange tea or barley tea is O.K. Generally, a pregnant woman should not drink a lot of tea."

## Cola, Coffee, Cocoa

Mr. Jung, a primary school teacher in Seoul, laments, "When my wife was pregnant with our first son, she enjoyed drinking Coca Cola everyday.

"As he was growing up, our boy's bones became fragile. A foot and an arm were broken twice when he was a baby. I thought this was caused by the Coke and other junk foods. Even now my son is very weak and is often beaten to tears by other children."

Naturally a mother would wish to avoid any beverages, no matter how tasty, which are potentially injurious to her baby's health.

According to some university students' mothers, the colorings of colas or coffee can filter through the placenta on down the umbilical cord to darken a baby's skin.

Worse than coloring, caffeine in coffee can impair a child's sensitive body and, particularly, his heart. Who hasn't witnessed how a few cups can disrupt a person's energy flow and send her through sleepless, emotional swings?

Seeing what just one glass of cocoa does to our over-active, ten-year-old daughter, I shudder at how such stimulants can affect a vulnerable fetus.

## What Shall Your Baby Eat?

A mother should feel joy when she sits down to eat (or starts to cook). This enhances the value of the food she sends to her companion at table.

Over the span of pregnancy, Mother should eat moderately. But, if she occasionally craves a special food (like strawberries) she can indulge a bit, or if she lacks appetite, she could accept this graciously. As a rule, one should choose food which is freshly grown or caught (fish), organic, and seasonal.

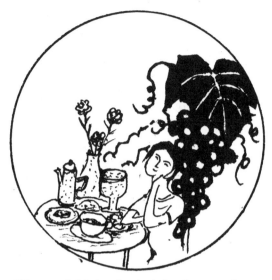

*I'll eat and drink only what's best for me* and *you.*

## Taboos

Lee Sa Ju Dang, in her *New Theory of Embryonic Education* (1801), says, "A pregnant woman should avoid the following foods:

Wormy, sour or crooked fruits; raw vegetables; cold rice; poorly cooked rice or meat; spoiled meat or fish; alcoholic beverages; donkey meat; scaleless fish; barley malt; garlic; yams; turnips; peaches; dog; rabbit; small crabs; mutton; chicken; duck; sparrow flesh; mushrooms; Job's Tears; cinnamon; deer; and foul-smelling foods."

Most of these are sensible prohibitions, based on centuries of experience, for avoiding an upset stomach or other unfortunate consequences of wrong food. Many taboos are due to the folk superstition of similarity, that "like begets like." For example, rabbit is omitted for fear of a hare-lip; crab could produce brittle bones; chicken, chicken flesh; duck, webbed toes; and sparrow, "a frivolous and undignified character."

Even if consumed by the father before conception, exotic foods could hurt a baby.

During our interview, Miss Yang, a middle school teacher, grows excited and says, "About twenty years ago, my uncle ate a bowl of snake soup, for stimulating his sexuality. Soon after, my aunt became pregnant and bore my girl cousin. Strangely enough, she was born with dry, scaly skin all over her body. It had a pink and white diamond pattern, like on a snake's skin!"

*"You're kidding!"*

"No, really! She's my cousin; I've seen it myself!"

Another schoolteacher, Mrs. Kim, concurs, "About fifty years ago, my father's brother died when he was only nine-years-old. Recently I came to know that my grandmother had eaten some dog-meat soup during her pregnancy, and that's why my uncle was born with an incurable disease."

*"You don't say!"*

## Fruit

Pregnant women in Asia crave fruit, especially if slightly sour. They favor apples, cherries, plums, strawberries, and watermelons, fresh in season. Oranges, however, are left out because they could produce an over-active child.

"Apples (in the morning)," my mother-in-law says, "grace a child with fair skin and rosy cheeks."

Ugly-colored or shaped fruits, however, can produce a "homely daughter."

"In India," says my neighbor, Professor Tulasi, "the craving for sour fruit is taken as a sign of pregnancy. The woman wishes to taste mango, raw or dry tamarind (a reddish sickle-shaped fruit), orange, or lemon. Papaya is not allowed, because it purges the body and can bring on a miscarriage."

Indonesian Professor Kentjono joins in, "Pregnant women in my country crave sour fruit, like green mangoes. Pineapple is forbidden due to its sharp character."

## Seeds and Nuts

"Walnuts," my mother-in-law says, "are good for the child's brain." My wife adds, "Black sesame cookies, since they need a lot of chewing, were eaten by Confucian scholars to stimulate their brains."

"Seeds feed your own seed (baby)" states Professor Pak Chon Guk, O.M.D., "so most (including nuts) are good for pregnant women. Black sesame seed is especially helpful, because it nourishes the kidneys. We say that 'the kidney is the seed of the human being.' Lotus and pine nuts are O.K. Sunflower seeds are forbidden, because they contain some poison."

Dr. Pak cautions, "Seeds and nuts are fatty, eating a lot isn't good for a pregnant woman."

## Vegetables

In the courts of the Choson Dynasty (1392–1910), a pregnant queen had to follow a very strict diet that emphasized foods made of a variety of pulses, vegetables, and seaweed, records Lee Won Sup in *The Royal Family's Teachings for Raising Life* (1993). He also explains in the newspaper article, "Prenatal Care and Diet of Choson Dynasty":

> Starting from the eighth month of pregnancy, she was nurtured intensively on beans with dishes such as bean soup, bean noodles, bean cake, and bean curd and made to drink the milk of a mountain sheep. The reason the queen dined on beans was that it ensured the baby's longevity and health, while sharpening its mind. It was a crucial task and great responsibility for the pregnant queen to eat a well-balanced diet.
>
> The Chinese character indicating the head(頭)includes the character meaning 'bean ( 豆 ).' As Chinese characters have symbolic meaning built into their structure, the Eastern sages made the character thousands of years ago in such a form knowing that the bean is necessary for cerebral growth.

Lee Jae Young, an old Taoist herbalist, points out, "Whereas fruit may have too much *yin* (cold and wet characteristics) and meat too much *yang* (hot and dry) energy, vegetables are the ideal food for humans, containing a good balance of *yin* and *yang*."

"Garlic makes the blood run fast; this can disturb the baby," warns Dr. Pak Chun Guk. "On the other hand, kidney-shaped beans are particularly beneficial for a pregnant woman, because they are shaped like embryos. Seeds also contain salt, though not in the Western sense."

"Ginseng is a very stimulating plant and can hurt a baby," says Dr. Jang Gi Nam. "It is generally taboo during pregnancy. (Ordinary table) salt can melt the placenta. Too much pepper can burn a hole in it."

For overall health, "Choose a variety of flavors," says Dr. Pak.

## Grains and Seafood

A pregnant Korean queen "consumed barley, carp, cow kidneys, and sea cucumber as special prenatal food in the early stages of pregnancy," explains Lee Won Sup in his article, "Prenatal Care and Diet of Choson Royalty."[9] "She was fed rice containing sliced radish with prawn, brown seaweed, and oyster during the middle stages of pregnancy. She was also made to consume millet, barley, and glutenous rice that had been steamed and dried three times, as well as abalone cooked in yellow loess."

Korean mothers claim, "Carp makes a child decent." Also, "A dish of sea cucumbers can heighten a child's intelligence. Anchovies can strengthen their bones." Young Im says, "A fish the size of your hand (or smaller) is nourishing; its calcium-rich bones are soft enough to grind in your teeth. It ought to be accompanied by a double-size portion of vegetables. Seaweed soup, however, is slippery, acts as a purgative, and so could bring on a miscarriage."

Still, an excess of fish can create problems for a baby. Dr. Sagan Ishizuka, the founder of Japanese "Macrobiotics," suffered from a lifelong skin disease, which, writes his disciple Herman Aihara in *Acid and Alkaline* (1970), was the result of a kidney ailment acquired in the womb. Dr. Ishizuka's mother ate "too many fish and spices during her pregnancy." A sign of this is itchiness or a rash. The cure is to refrain.

"Spicy and salty food make the character of the baby tough and wild," Koreans believe. "Soft and mild dishes are best."

## Meat

The pregnant queen was discouraged from eating meat, since it was believed to have a "killing *ch'i*," dangerous for a baby.

According to Michio Kushi in Macrobiotic Pregnancy and Care of the Newborn (1984), indulging in red meat and fat is likely to affect the character of a pregnant woman's child, causing him to be "head-strong" like an ox, or perhaps "hot-tempered" like a bull.

Still, a Korean woman often treats herself to a meal of well-steamed, thinly sliced pork (with plenty of sour, water *kimchi*) towards term. Professor Pak says, "Pork nourishes the kidneys. It is a seed food and salty." It cools down the body, giving the woman strength for enduring labor, and perhaps a little oil for helping her baby slide out more easily!

## Desserts

During the Choson Dynasty, a pregnant queen would be cautioned not to eat a lot of sweets, because they could "soften the baby's brain." Sugar is addictive for mother and child both, Miss Goh, a girl student, affirms. "My mother craved ice cream when bearing me, so now my favorite food is ice cream!"

## Table Manners

"When my grandmother was expecting her first child," Miss Yoon, a university student, reports, "my great-grandmother took it upon herself to enforce a rigorous code of fetal training on the expectant mother, as well as on the rest of the household.

"She informed her daughter-in-law that a woman with-child should be particularly mindful of her every thought and act, because this is important for the future well-being of her baby. Consequently, my grandmother was told that she should not eat from any chipped bowls or plates, and that all fruits should be cut in such a way that there would be no sharp angles, only curves (for this is also for shaping the baby's body and mind)."

"My grandmother used to tell us, 'Eat with good fortune.' This means that our life will be reflected in the way in which we take our food. If we have polite manners and good habits while eating, these will carry over to other activities, bringing us good luck."

## Magical Flavor

Imagine,

*walking over to apple trees spread out on the hills.*

*A doe scampers away, a few apples drop off a tree, bouncing with the sounds of galloping hooves.*

*Pick one up, feel its coolness, discern its color, sniff it, and famished, nibble into its crispy, juicy freshness.*

## Chinese Beauties in the Park

One summer's day in 1993, while roaming about Sun Yat Sen Park in Taichung, Taiwan, brushing aside the leafy strands of a willow, I come upon a beautiful woman with black, silky hair, seated in the center of a curving, white-stone bench. She is heavy with new life and fatigued from carrying it around in the heat. In a slight breeze from waters behind her, and under the shade of the willows, she rests, the folds of her flower-patterned maternity dress hanging loosely.

I approach with my camera, indicating through a smile that I'd like to take her picture. But she smiles shyly and, lifting a hand over her face, turns aside. If I persist, perhaps I will offend the "precious" one in her womb. Indeed, it is out of concern for his or her well-being that she has turned aside from a stranger and kept her protecting body's image away from the admiration or envy of unknown, blue eyes. I would be a hypocrite to insist, so I smile understandingly and leave her alone with her child.

Unable to resist, however, a few minutes later I return to the spot, but she is gone. Just her memory remains on the empty chair. So I take a picture of that and also draw a rough sketch of her from memory.

A little after, she crosses over the white footbridge, a dutiful husband by her side, his supporting hand under her arm.

*   *   *

Before departing Taiwan, I linger a few days at a Buddhist temple on Lion's Head Mountain. Everywhere on my trip, I have been encountering pregnant women in their ample, flowery dresses. Even the receptionist at the temple lodging house is well along in pregnancy. She is tall, has short-cropped black hair, and smiles at me warmly as if recognizing that I am a friend. She even guides me up a steep flight of stairs to show me the washroom, the dining-room, and where I was to sleep. The climb does not weary her; movement and fresh air is, indeed, good for pregnancy and future labor. I marvel at her graceful carriage and good cheer.

Soon I take a walk up the mountain and, as I pass under an orange-painted, wooden archway, another pregnant woman appears, also tall, but with long, brownish hair. She smiles at me spontaneously, flashing her clean, white teeth. I am intoxicated by my good fortune and gaze in wonder as she passes by and down the numerous low, winding stairs. I am being charmed by the pregnant women of the world.

All around is green, bountiful vegetation. A light blue and black, long-tailed butterfly flutters about my head. Cicadas click in chorus on the branches of trees, and sweet perfume from flowers floats down the mountain, surrounding me with an invisible womb. I climb the mountain, winding up the numerous low, moss green steps where the woman had recently been. Surely the birth she would give a few months from now would be a comparatively easy one. The child born would be one of beauty, one with an eye, nose, and ear for the wonders of nature.

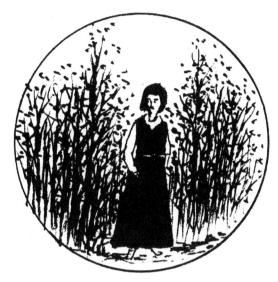

*We go slowly through the fields of tranquility.*

## Observing Oneself in Water

Imagine,

*crossing halfway over an arching bridge, with the sun sliding over your shoulders. Observe being in water, the drifting sky blue or pink of a maternity dress.*

*Note the mirrored yellow green and orange showers of maple leaves wafting over the eddies.*

*Gaze up through the transparent colors of the leaves and trace the veins, like rivers with tiny, branching tributaries.*

*Peer down through crystalline waters to the minnows, their shadows darting over quartz and feldspar pebbles, alongside bits of mica lying in the sand.*

*Your child gains eyes for the beauty of life.*

*Raindrops are tapping here and there on leaves, even on your hair and cheeks....*

*Go on touching seeds, stems, buds, leaves, flowers, and fruits...; of course, feel the belly, and your own fruit stirring.*

*Once born, (s)he'll recall and continue to cherish the beauty of touch.*

*Surround yourself with fresh air and flowering herbs; tell the baby, "smell these gardenias..., and some lilies...."*

*Step now, into the small woods, where the sight is dim, save for an occasional twinkling star, or a greenish gold firefly blinking over the trees.*

*At last, the cock "coquries," the cuckoo "sukoos," doves "coo," and small birds cry out, one species after the other, heralding a new day.*

## Strolling with a Companion

One spring day in 1976, I hesitantly called on Audrey, a British woman, eight-months pregnant, in her Kyoto, Japan house:

> *"What if*
> *she trips*
> *down*
>
> > *her*
> > *winding*
> > *steps*
>
> > > *on*
> > > *the way*
> > > *to greet*
> > > *me*                          *and Baby*
> > > *pops out...!?"*
>
> > > > *But she's*
> > > > *careful,*
> > > > *at ease....*

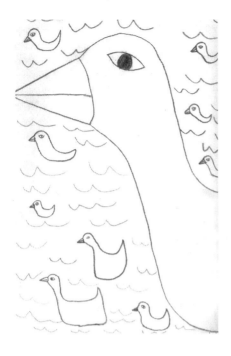

*I'll carry you through the waters of life
as gracefully as a swan.*

Drawing by Chalina Seligson.

Now I recall my friends, as they were then, the young British couple, twenty-five years ago in Kyoto: Audrey is near term. Her husband drives to the countryside. They step out of the car ahead of me. At sunset, they stroll arm in arm, on a smooth, tree-lined path. All around is fresh air, moss, ferns, crickets chirruping under colorful maple leaves, and birds chirping, snuggling up in trees for the night, as if in an Eden.

It is desirable for an expecting woman to carry a baby gracefully, from the center of gravity in her belly, like a swan. As she sways, so does Baby. His or her body will shift to such rhythms after birth.

## A Good-Hearted Person

In her *New Theory of Embryonic Education*, Lee Sa Ju Dang recommends that a pregnant woman, in her passage through the waters of life, avert her eyes from disconcerting sights, including, "a mask,

43

a clown, a dwarf, a monkey, jesting, a quarrel, a punishment, a murder, any injury to others, a deformed person, a person with a grave disease, a rainbow, thunder, lightning, a shooting star, a comet, an ill-boding star, an eclipse, a flood, a fire, a tree snapping in two, a house collapsing, copulations of birds or beasts, and creeping insects." If the mother gets caught up in such a gloomy, violent, lewd or other disturbing sight, it could "injure her child's spirit" or even touch off a miscarriage.

This is why Sa Ju Dang advises that, in order to safeguard one's body and also to influence the child's disposition, a woman ought to direct her eyes to sights of beauty and character, such as "a noble man, a good-hearted person, a white or clear gem, a peacock, bright and beautiful objects, the sayings of the sages hanging from scrolls, a Taoist ascetic, a court official's uniform, and jade ornaments."

## Seeing a Child

Imagine,

*serenely strolling along a seacoast, feeling the waves wash over your toes, cradling, and murmuring to, a gleeful child in Mother's (or Father's) arms.*

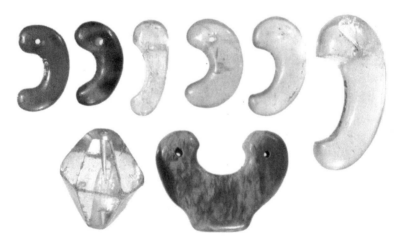

*Jade, agate, and crystal embryos (Three Kingdoms Period, post-688, Gyeongju National Museum, Korea)*

# Caressing a Jade Child

*On*
*the*
*way*

*we*
*bore*

*a*
*girl*

*comma*
*on*
*the*
*silk*
*worm's*
*neck*
*(facing*
*West)*

*she*
*grew*

*into*

*a*
*fairy*

*Also*

*we*
*bore*

*a*
*son*

*comma*
*on*
*the*
*silk*
*worm's*
*neck*
*(facing*
*East)*

*he*
*grew*
*into*

*an*
*angel.*

Jade commas of various colors: blood red, bone white, egg yellow streaked with turquoise, blue gray flecked by pink, gold and purple clouds, each containing a blackened hole near the top where you might imagine an eye to be on an embryo, hanging from colorfully beaded necklaces.... Some of the commas are as small as a baby's fingernail, and others larger than my thumb.

Marveling at them during a visit to a museum in Ueno Park, Tokyo, in early 1989, it strikes me, having seen similar ones at the Imperial Museum in Taipei, and at the National Museum in Seoul,

45

that these comma-shaped jade ornaments wrought long ago, are images of hoped for babies—embryos hanging on gold umbilical strings from the crowns and belts of kings, as well as the earrings and necklaces of queens. I try to imagine their migrations from royal hand to hand, overland from China to Korea, overseas to Japan.

The jade embryos are attached to prayers addressed to heavenly deities for the conception of royal sons and daughters, and for the repopulation of realms where countless have died from generations of war, starvation, and disease: prayers for the children of gods to be reincarnated on Earth. To me, the commas look like ears, too; tiny ones by which to hear the sound of Heaven's voice. Charming ears dangling from the crown, earlobes, throat, and waist, by which to call the spirits of Heaven to the bodies of kings and queens.

Jades worn on clothing or warmly grasped in Mother's hand were also employed for nurturing the embryo in the impregnated, royal womb. I stand long, wondering at the glass-contained embryos. Their magic is now stored away and forgotten, yet I strive to revive and set it to work at its ancient purposes.

A pregnant queen, relates Lee Won Sup in his article, "Prenatal Care and Diet of Choson Royalty," "would gaze for a long time at items made of jade such as ornamental hairpins, trinkets, girdles, and twin rings to visually aid the emotional and character formation of the fetus. The effect of the color of jade, sea green, was believed to reach the fetus through the eyes of the queen and benefit its emotional cultivation. Also, a pine forest was constructed in the secret garden of the palace so that the queen could gaze at it habitually for the benefit of the fetus.

"The eunuch in charge of making the royal liquor always conducted a rite of offering in the initial stage of making the yeast. On such an occasion, he always dressed in a jade-colored robe. The idea behind this practice was that the microscopic yeast like the jade color very much.

"Hence the belief that the fetus would favor the jade color in the initial stages of cellular development during the ten (lunar) months of pregnancy. The queen, during her prenatal training, also fully dressed in jade-colored clothes from her robe on down to her shoes and accessories."[10]

Miss Yu, a Korean student, reports, "In the way of our ancestors, at first, a pregnant woman decides full-heartedly to do good for her baby. Then, she will often clasp a piece of beautifully colored jade in her hand. Surely every woman enjoys doing this, but we should know why. Whenever the jade-processing artist is concentrating on its clarity and color, he grinds the precious stone with a feeling softer than skin. For this reason, it is said that the color of jade is not made of the sun, but of the moon. Moreover, the mysterious color of jade has a delicate and miraculous quality for the little baby's future life. To touch a beautiful piece of jade as often as possible yields the good fruit of raising our human mind to a higher level."

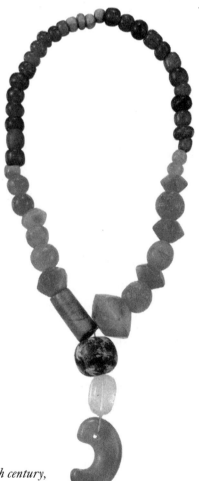

For a craftsman to carve the finest jade, he must have a continuously calm and caring heart and a precise touch. He must be master of himself, and not a slave to outer stimuli, because with one flighty thought and slip of the fingers, the jewel can be ruined. In the same way is a woman encouraged to give single-minded fidelity to the precious child in her womb, keeping it pure and round, bright and free.

*Jade embryo necklace (Silla Kingdom Fifth–Sixth century, Gyeongju National Museum, Korea)*

# A Virtuous Woman's Story

In *A Loyal and Virtuous Woman's Story,* Lu Hiang (first century A.D.) says, "When Queen Ta Jen *(Great Responsibility)* was pregnant, her eyes looked on no improper sight, her ears listened to no licentious sound, and her lips uttered no word of pride.

"When the King (Wen) was born, he was intelligent and sage, so that when his mother taught him one thing, he learned a hundred things, and in the end he became the founder of the Chou dynasty."

His wife, Queen Ta Jen, said, "I took care of my behavior and cleaned my heart, so that I was able to bear a great person (King Woo)."

Both queens are celebrated in the classic *Book of Odes:*

*Pure and reverent was Ta Jen,*
*The mother of King Wen;*

*Loving was she to Chou Chiang—*
*a wife becoming the House of Chou.*

*Ta Ssu inherited her excellent fame,*
*and from her came a hundred sons.*[11]

"A hundred sons" refers to the many generations of children to be influenced by Ta Jen's and Ta Ssu's conscientious behavior, and perhaps this was more important to them than the limited goal of nurturing only one son. In fact, the whole of China and its neighboring countries, kings and noblemen, scholars and artists, and millions of other people for over three thousand years, through the medium of their own mothers, have received the touch of Queen Ta Jen's and Ta Ssu's wise, compassionate pregnancies. From this, we can begin to appreciate the great influence that one woman could have by being single-heartedly devoted to her unborn child. And, Queen Jin's considerate teachings continue, spreading with Chinese, Korean, and Japanese women to cultures around the world. One day, with the migrations of human beings beyond our Earth, they shall sail to other stars.

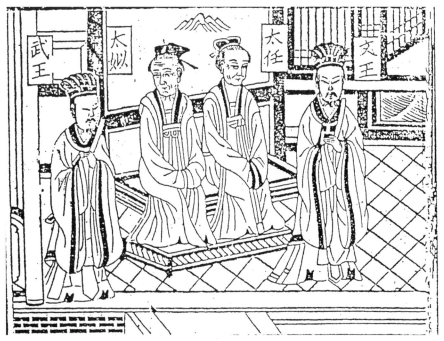

*From left to right, King Wu, his mother Queen Sze, her mother-in-law Queen Jin, and her son King Wan on a page from the Chinese classic*
A Loyal and Virtuous Woman's Story *by Lew Heang, 130 A.D.*

A common saying is, "The (moral) root of the empire is the root of the nation, the root of the nation is the family, and the root of the family is the person." Still, the root of the person is the embryo in the womb.

## Teacher of Responsibility

*She stands in the blue and endless sea. The water is calm and crystalline. All of a sudden, a glittering woman appears, crying out to her, dancing.*

*Sim Sa Im Dang can only glance at her because of the astonishing brightness all around, but she supposes that the lady is an angel, one who is wearing such wondrous clothing that Sa Im Dang faints.*

*A little later, recovering her senses, she glances over at the angel, who*

49

*is slowly approaching. She is carrying a baby whose skin is white and clean.*

*Smiling, she comes up to Sa Im Dang, hands her the baby, and leaves without a word. The baby is healthy and fat, a boy. Sa Im Dang sets him tenderly on her breast. The angel disappears into the sea.*

Upon awaking, she realizes that she is pregnant: "A god has given my body a baby to raise into the world."

Sa Im Dang knows that the child might not reach its potential for glory, which the dream suggested, if she doesn't assist it. What is received congenitally, must be supplemented by acquired characteristics, and for this, she is particularly gifted.

From an early age, Sa Im Dang had been a student of the Chinese classics, a sensitive poetess, and a masterful painter of nature, especially of flowers and insects, in both the folk and Chinese traditions. All of these qualities from her everyday life were already on hand to fruitfully influence the child in her womb: her delicate, discerning taste was transmitted to the fetus through her feelings, thoughts, and actions.

According to Oh Shi Rim's *Shin Sa Im Dang and Child Education* (1988), after conceiving, "Sa Im Dang took good care of her body. She would not eat strange foods or look at unpleasant sights. She refrained from evil thoughts and foul language. And, she prayed to Heaven to, 'Give me a great baby, like King Wen of China.'"

Her self-chosen name shares the character *Im* or *Jin* (任), meaning *Responsibility*, with King Wen's mother, Queen Jin, the Chinese founder of *Embryonic Education.*

Sa Im Dang sojourned to her parents' house to await delivery of the baby. Her mother cared for her during those weeks and would assist with the birth.

As the day approached, Sa Im Dang poured some water into a basin and carried it reverently to the bedside for bathing her expected baby. Just before giving birth, she dozed in a small room and dreamt:

*During a storm, amidst great winds, a black dragon rises up out of the sea. It flies into the sky and approaches me. I flee, but it follows me into a room inside my parents' house.*

*The dragon, filling up the room with its body, sits down and stares at her. She feels pain and wakes up.*

She told her dream to her mother, who responded, "This baby is bound to be a great person in the future, so please take care of him with all of your heart."

Sa Im Dang strove to make her thoughts cleaner and brighter than those of others. Her neighbors said, "She absorbed the spirits of Heaven, Truth, and Knowledge until nothing else remained in her mind, allowing her to produce a son such as Yul Guk."

Yi Yul Guk, (born 1536), grew up to become a Neo-Confucian philosopher of the highest rank, an accomplished poet, and a government cabinet minister (at various times) of War, Education, and Economy. He has been cherished for his penetrating insight, fairness, and loyal character to this day. These qualities have been attributed to the pure and artistic nature of his mother's behavior during and following her pregnancy.

## Teacher of the Unborn Child

Lee Sa Ju Dang, "whose virtue spread like a fragrance to her village," claims in her *New Theory of Embryonic Education*, that "a man's good character originates in Heaven, but his dispositions are developed by his parents. The former is inborn; and the latter, acquired. A habitual disposition is hard to give up, so a pregnant woman must be discreet in her behavior.

"She must not harm anyone or even entertain thoughts of killing animals or playing tricks on others. She should not be sly, jealous, greedy, deceitful, thieving, or envious of anyone superior. Nor should she interrupt another's words or slander others. She should be mindful of her gestures when annoyed, avoid scolding or manipulating others, whispering gossip, talking frivolously, or meddling unnecessarily in the affairs of others." Otherwise, "a mother's exasperation can sicken the child's blood. A dastardly act can drain its vitality." Finally, "A jealous or hateful mind does not bring fortune, but a comfortable and smiling person is always lucky."

Doctors Che Sam Sup, O.M.D., and Pak Chon Guk, O.M.D., in their commentary on the *New Theory* concur that, "If, as a result of complicated affairs occurring in a household, the mother has insecure feelings and becomes fussy in her behavior, the baby, too, will be born with a finicky disposition, not a generous one.

"On the other hand, if the mother is gracious in her assessment of others and considerate in serving her own parents, her baby will grow up doing the same."

A folk belief adds, "If you conceive a dislike for someone, your baby will be born resembling that person."

So, Lee Sa Ju Dang declares, "A sick person can be cured by medicines, but a fetus only by his mother's 'heart.'"

An old Korean medical text written by Haw Jun, *The Eastern Medical Treasury* (1610), asks a pregnant woman not to take offense or get angry under any circumstances. Whenever she is angry, *ch'i* rises up to her head and stays there until she recovers her stability. As a result, that energy is diverted from nourishing the baby in her womb.

## A Beautiful Smile

Simply smiling can overcome feelings of gloom:

*Concentrate on, and feel your heart softening and opening; feel grateful for being alive.*

*After a while, raise this sensation on up your throat, then your lips.*

*Let Mother's (Father's) eyes shine blissfully down through to the adorable baby.*

## Spreading Joy to the World

*Off the curving beach of Thailand, the water is as clear as lime jello, coming in tiny waves.*

*We let our one-year-old Chalina slide between us and sink into the cool water.*

*About a foot below, she begins paddling her arms and legs.*

*"She's swimming...!" Young Im exclaims.*

*"Yes, really...; she must've learned in the womb!"*

*"But she only knows how to swim underwater!"*

*"We'd better pull her up...."*

One afternoon, I ask our Chinese dinner guest, Wang Su Yi, who is eight-months pregnant, "Can you feel your baby swimming around in the womb?"

"Oh yes, but it's more like dancing, modern dancing; he's kicking and waving his arms."

"When did you first begin to feel him inside?"

"At about five months."

"Was he dancing then?"

"No, from five to about seven months I just felt he was present. There would be a sudden movement or sensation and I'd think, 'He's happy,' or else, 'He's angry.'"

"What was the difference between feeling that he was angry or happy?"

"I can't say for sure; it was more that I felt as if he was feeling just like I did at the moment. Now when I'm angry, he dances about more, kicking and punching. When I'm happy, he also feels gentler, at ease."

The other guest at our table, Mrs. Joó Young Suk, a Korean primary school teacher, puts in, "I have a friend who, when pregnant, wasn't getting along with her mother-in-law and suffered a lot from stress because of it. At last, she bore a son.

"Recently she said to me, 'As my boy grows up, he becomes more impatient and gets angry more readily. Maybe this is because I wasn't able to take it easy during pregnancy.'"

My wife Young Im illustrates how a mother's compulsive thoughts and behavior during pregnancy can influence her child's development:

"When my mother was newly married, my father gave her a camel-hair coat as a gift. In those days of the Japanese Occupation

(1910–1945), it was a rare possession, so a cousin used to cast envious glances at it whenever my mother wore it.

"When my mother accompanied my father, who was a mining engineer, to his camp in the mountains, she left her camel-hair coat at home, since it wasn't fair for the poorly-paid miners to see. A few months later, she returned home and opened her clothes chest to get her coat out but was shocked to find it missing. She suspected her cousin, who was pregnant at the time, but said nothing.

"A couple of months later, her cousin gave birth to a son, but over the years he grew up to be a petty thief. None of our relatives felt comfortable with his visiting their homes."

A study of juvenile delinquents at a local reform school, reported in a Seoul newspaper, suggests that their maladjustment to society is linked "to having received no *Embryonic Education.*"

It is also common these days to read in Seoul papers of complaints by monks and educators that "today's rise in juvenile crime is due to a lack of *Embryonic Education.*"

Originally, a child is neither "good" nor "bad," but rather "pure," as the Balinese say, "close to Heaven." In the womb, (s)he is in a state of absolute openness, unable to distinguish between "right and wrong" or "you and me." A mother's (even a father's) feelings and accompanying behavior during pregnancy are contagious and can influence the child's dispositions in one direction or the other.

## Ways of Loving-Kindness

Kim Jo Shin, a Korean sage, counsels,

"Never forget the existence of your baby. Always send it respect and love with your silent (telepathic) heart. Always try to feel what it wants."

Following the ways of predecessors, conscientious Asian women are poring over magazine articles and books on *Embryonic Education.* They are realizing that it is possible to raise themselves up to higher levels of self-understanding. They are developing an appreciation for the joys of living in the present moment, as well as a calm sense of the healing cycles of time in order to create comfortable conditions for the child in the womb.

Some pray to the object of their faith, for their hearts to be cleansed of malicious thoughts, not only for the strength and benevolence to take care of their own child, but also for the needy ones of strangers.

Some chant before altars of burning candles and incense, or sit with freshly-washed bodies, contemplating uplifting spiritual passages, or else meditatively noting the rising and passing of each comforting or disturbing thought and emotion until they reach clarity and serenity.

Some practice forgiveness of wrongdoers, as well as mercy for all creatures, sparing even insects or leaves of grass (perhaps these women sense the mysterious workings of *karma*—that others will, in turn, care for them in times of need; or else, they are afraid of transferring a cruel character to their baby).

Some overcome selfishness by performing acts of charity with feelings of loving-kindness, offering alms, food, or clothing to the needy.

Some engage in the arts, such as flower gardening, decorative sewing, water-color painting, or calligraphy. Such activities beautify a mother and baby's mind. So does reciting favorite poems, playing an instrument, or singing joyously.

All in all, good parenting comes down to practicing not only clean manners, but also how to love. Love is giving of oneself, not desiring to possess another. Love is fidelity and mutual trust. Love is found in small, intimate glances and acts; in gifts like a touch, a kiss, a word of encouragement; a glance at the sun, moon, or stars. Love is not from the desire to have, but rather in the inclination to serve others out of inherent goodness. Gentleness, devotion, and compassion: all are gifts of love.

Love is like the sun, casting light freely on your child and all about you. It is the ultimate charity.

## Chinese Looking-Glass Meditation

*Close your eyes, effortlessly breathing from the circle of the womb …*

*Quietly let thoughts disappear, seeing the curve of your eyebrows and the outline of your lips as if in a mirror …*

*Say humbly,*

*"Baby, we're so grateful you're here with us."*

## Colors for a Young Artist

One afternoon, Young Im leafs through *JAM JAM,* a Korean women's magazine (October 1990), translating an intriguing interview: Mrs. Shin Mi Jae, O.M.D., claims that, "All matter, including rocks, trees, animals, and humans, have their origin in *ch'i* (bio-energy) or the gradually concretizing forms of light and color.

"By learning to clearly visualize separate colors and, afterwards, to manipulate them into various shapes and images, a mother's (or father's) heart will gain flexibility and strength. It will begin to approach the creative ways of 'original nature,' and this can benefit her baby's developing emotions and intelligence.

"The more vividly and intricately the mother is able to compose pictures in her mind's self-luminous 'eye,' the more textually rich life will appear around her and the stronger she will feel. Even her dreams will become more colorful and fine."

During her own pregnancy, Dr. Shin practiced visualizing and manipulating into forms the Five Colors of changing nature. Along with other *Embryonic Education* techniques, she achieved admirable results for her forthcoming daughter. I become acquainted with the clear-eyed two-year-old after being greeted by Dr. Shin at her downtown Seoul clinic.

Dr. Shin says, "I advise my pregnant patients to relax and gaze meditatively at a *colorogram* for ten minutes each day.

"Sky blue represents Wood (or Wind), growth, and aspiration.

"Rose red stands for Fire and warm open-hearted love.

"Sun yellow is the Earth and 'mind-spirit (soul).'

"White gold is Metal, foundation and harvest, cleanliness and health.

"Jet black is Water, the connection with our ancestors, night, gentle sex, deep-relaxed sleep.

"All these colors are interconnected, so a pregnant woman should contemplate their individual meanings, as well as the relationships as a whole."

\*    \*    \*

You can construct a *colorogram*[12] with colored paper, or watercolors on shiny white poster-board:

Draw a circle, fourteen inches in diameter, around another circle of eight inches.

Paint the inner circle sun yellow. Divide the outer circle into four equal portions: top, bottom, left, and right.

Paint the upper part (North), jet black; the right side (East) sky blue; the lower part (South), rose red; and the left side (West), white gold (or leave it white). Apply only bright, living colors, not dull ones.

What has been produced is a map of Creation.

You can contemplate it upon waking in the morning and before sleeping by:

*Considering individual colors and their relationships.*

*Allowing the field of vision to encompass the whole colorogram at once.*

*Bathing in the colors.*

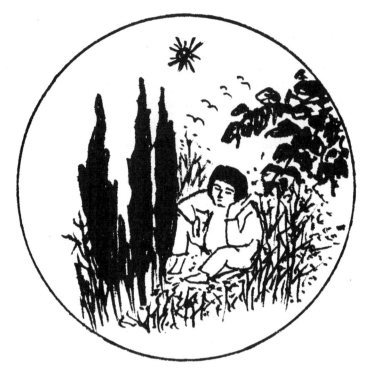

*In Nature's garden, let's linger, at peace.*

As an experiment, I have just stepped outside and gazed a few minutes each at the clear blue of the sky, the pink of a garage wall, the green of a house roof, and the yellow of autumn leaves—just the colors—with an otherwise empty mind.

Wow! I don't think I've ever seen color intensified like this before—even my myopia seems to have improved!

See the cloud-like particles of energy inside. One's mind can shape and color them at will, forming images. Practice gathering the light into a ball and then dispersing it again.

*Sit, at ease, facing South.*

*Move the eyes around slowly to fill in vibrant shapes and colors of these …*

## Dream Birds on Parade

*Misty gray, three-dimensional birds are strutting about on grass: a peacock from the East, a flamingo from the South, a golden eagle in the Center, a swan from the West, and a black crane from the North.*

If you can see them one at a time, then all moving and nodding together, you have begun painting with the "hands" of your "mind's eye"; having have taken formless *ch'i*, separated light from shadow, divided it into various colors, condensed it, and molded it into apparently "living" creatures. What's more, you can share these keys of creativity with your child.

"The forms and patterns a pregnant woman constructs in her imagination can possibly travel on light waves into her baby's mind," my neighbor Ed Button, a nuclear physicist, speculates.

## Animals on Parade

Now, sit comfortably, close your eyes, and visualize the following animals of light:

*Ambling through the eastern woodlands, a bright blue bear* (soothes your liver).

*Galloping under the southern sun, a rosy pony* (heart).

*Grazing in the surrounding savannah, a sun yellow cow* (spleen).

*Waddling up a western mountain, a bright white elephant* (lungs).

*Lapping from a northern stream, a shiny black deer* (kidneys).

You can take control of life and choose what to view on the outside or within the imagination, rather than becoming a victim of sexual or violent images and bright, flashing lights, such as those normally found on T.V. or in videos. The more alert your own senses become, the more you will appreciate the quiet, clear, but marvelous potentials of your universe, and, as a consequence, the more likely you can pass on creative, rather than destructive qualities to your child.

## A Labyrinth of Flowers

This is a journey for a mother and her small companion to enjoy. In fantasy,

*Stroll on a mossy path by petite blue and white flowers, ferns, and ivy, over rolling hills, under cherry trees blossoming into the soft hollows of a valley.*

*See storks wading in lotus ponds, and a stone wall strung by purple and white morning glories. Cross a foot-bridge arching into a palace with star and crescent-moon-shaped windows.*

*Winding hallways are lined with paintings of mothers and children. Soft-carpeted floors are covered with maroon and creamy peonies, and birds of paradise. On silk curtains, the sun and full moon, snow-clouded mountains, gushing waterfalls, and fresh pines appear.*

*Cherubs, with bugles and harps, flutter about a glass dome.*

*Your smiling spouse offers a welcome embrace.*

## Songs for a Young Musician

Chinese music was prescribed to shape the soul of a royal child in the womb. Ching Ssu (quoted by Ja Hee, 130 B.C.) in *The Truth of Embryonic Education from Ancient Times*, explains:

When the king's wife has been pregnant for seven months, she goes to reside in a special house. A professional musician joins her there and plays for her. He keeps his instrument in the house and awaits the queen's orders. If she wants to hear music, he must play only what is appropriate for her condition. If it isn't suitable, he should be ordered to stop.

During the last three months of pregnancy, the musician must play music only to the queen's liking.

When the son of the king is born and cries, the musician makes correct music, integrating the crying sounds with those of the strings in a composition.

As the crown prince heard his own cries incorporated into musical notes, they had a soothing effect. One function of court music was to evoke harmonious feelings, influencing the child's and his mother's dispositions. Its objects were joy, serenity, and grace. Ladies in the Tang courts used to step in rhythm to the music of the day, and designated melodies were played to inform them of various duties or to call them to the king's audience hall.

A distinctive style of music, displaying dignity and grandeur, was danced to elegantly during ceremonies, and this reflected sounds naturally given off by (gods in) Heaven. It bore melodies, like that of great rivers and mountains, or swirls of clouds, and of stars, which flowed on and on. When earthly beings played such songs, their petitions and prayers could float up to the compliant ears of Heaven.

From Lee Won Sup's *The Royal Family's Teachings for Raising Life* (1993), we learn that music was played in Korea during the Choson Dynasty (1392–1910) to calm the queen and cultivate her baby in the womb. "Music was prescribed to create a quiet environment for the queen in her chambers. Stately court music was played on the *kayagum* and *komungo* (zither-like instruments) for the baby at daybreak or at night just before the queen went to sleep, with the aim of stimulating the brain development of the fetus and cultivating his healthy emotional and moral character, but flute music was omitted because it could stir up the mother's emotions. Music was an education for a soft, mild manner and calm intelligence, not only for enjoyment."

In a traditional Seoul teahouse, over a cup of green tea, Mrs Hong, a primary school teacher, tells my wife and me: "I have two daughters. The eldest one, to whom I failed to give much thought or care during pregnancy, is now very restless and frequently gets angry. The younger one, for whom I kept the rules (of *Embryonic Education*), is more calm and mild-mannered. For her, I purposely played classical music, especially Antonio Vivaldi's *The Four Seasons*."

A woman's living situation, the state of her mind and body, varies each day of a pregnancy. Every child conceived is molded, accordingly, by the nature of turmoil and/or tranquility the mother is experiencing. The child's disposition is not just a matter of genetics or of chance but can be influenced, as here, for example, by the music its mother hears.

"What a baby hears is not what its parent hears," my physicist neighbor, Ed Button, Ph.D., emphasizes. "Sound waves are amplified in the amniotic fluid of the womb."

Fancy being in a child's place, and what he would prefer to be hearing at such a delicate stage—the soft hum of a harp-string or

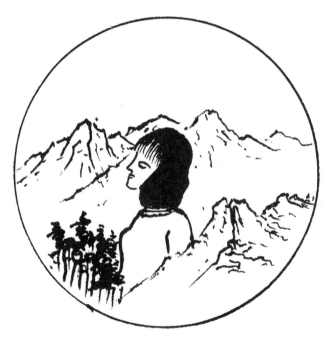

*Let's pause and listen to the symphony of the stream.*

the clash of cymbals. An unborn child is helpless, unable to filter out fast, loud, or other potentially disturbing sounds. Commercials, for example, can disrupt an expecting woman's, and consequentially, her baby's, peace of mind.

Albeit, if she stays calm in the face of disturbing sounds, her baby will more likely remain so, too. She is his measure of safety. If she maintains a pleasant feeling, it can carry over.

## Sounds of Natural Growth

"Modern pop music has too much Fire for a mother and unborn baby to absorb," claims Kim Do Hyang, a popular Korean singer and composer of thirty CD's of *Embryonic Education* music,[13] following the Five Phases (Water, Wood, Fire, Earth, and Metal) of development in nature.

In 1994, I chanced upon a lecture given by the traditionally dressed, bearded Mr. Kim at the Inner World Cultural Center in Seoul and upon making his acquaintance, asked, "Could you explain more about your prenatal music?"

"Of course. This music is for Mother and Baby both. It makes them peaceful and harmonizes their *ch'i,* or vital power, by means of the flow of sound waves through their bodies. Since mother and baby are a unit, the condition of one affects the other.

In the West, the focus is on the development of the baby's body. Here we focus on *ch'i* and the relationship of sound wave energy to the various organs.

There are five phases of development of the organs, each one divided into two parts and each of these requiring a different combination of sound waves. This can be understood through an analogy of the changes in the body to the changes of the seasons.

During the first month, when the Liver *(ch'i),* and the second, when the Gall Bladder *(ch'i)* is beginning to grow, various Wood sound waves are played. Castanets can produce Wood sounds, for example, but they can also make Fire. The flow of the energy is like Spring with the plants growing up and up.

The next phase is Fire. This is related to the Heart and Small Intestine during the third and fourth months. Fire sounds correspond to Summer when the leaves are getting rounder and wider.

This is followed by Soil. It concerns the Spleen and Stomach in the fifth and sixth months. Soil is related to Late Summer, like a long, rainy day. The sound is like that of a yellow color; it is deep and wide as a valley's echo.

Next is the Iron phase. This has to do with the Lungs and Large Intestine during the seventh and eighth months. Iron corresponds to Autumn. The sounds are more hot, like of trees bearing fruit.

After this is the Water phase. It relates to the Kidneys and Bladder in the ninth and tenth months. It's like Winter with the sounds of everything settling down, down.

There are various kinds of sounds for each phase; for example, Water has that of a river flowing and rain falling. Although both Kidneys and Bladder are related to Water, different Water sounds are appropriate for each of them, following the ideas of *yin* and *yang*, that is, plus and minus, or greater and lesser, making a whole.

We use bird songs, too, but various ones can be like Wood, Fire, Soil, Iron, or Water and so fit different phases of pregnancy. The same goes for other nature sounds.

From the standpoint of Oriental Medicine, we look at how the flow of *ch'i* affects the baby's growth. (1) We influence the power of *ch'i* through sound waves. (2) And, the sounds move like a melody, affecting both inner and outer development. (3) Our music is calming to both mother and child, like a meditation. So, by this process, the mother is relaxed, and the sounds assist the baby's and mother's bodily development.

We're already getting news about the first babies, who are now about ten-months old. Many mothers have called in, about one hundred of them, and when we ask them, 'What is the difference between your other babies and this one?' they say, 'This one is more peaceful and when he is crying, if I play the music for him again, he stops and goes back to sleep.'

I tell them, 'This is only the beginning; wait ten or twenty years and then you will see what a fine child you have, how mild-mannered and brilliant.'

Now our music is being tested by doctors in America at Johns Hopkins University."

A parent can send a child sounds of birds, streams, and breeze-blown leaves; the music of nature. Also, she can offer her a "music of serenity," which emanates from the heart, calmly sounding, now and again throughout a day.

## Singing One's Song

*Sit, breathing freely; accept air, and let go.*

*Place hands lightly over your baby; feel the womb rising and falling.*

*Take in a breath, then sing out vowels (A, E, I, O, U) one at a time, up and down the scale.*

*Compose songs without (or with) words, following the course of your feelings.*

*Serenade your baby, as if a lover outside his window.*

*Dance (gently) to your song.*

## Garden of Pregnancy Dreams

To a baby in the womb paradise, the mother is the sparkling goddess within whom all of his waking and sleeping life revolves. It's a flattering, but also a tremendous and, at times, frightening responsibility. She is often groping in the dark, not knowing the condition of her child or what to do about it. She may feel it is simply best to let her follow a natural course. Nature will care for the baby and there is little she can do.

In most cases, she may be right. If she goes about her life with feelings and acts of devoted, maternal love, she will most likely turn out to become a fine, loving person. But this might not be so if the circumstances of her waking life and nightmares combine to create an emotionally charged atmosphere, abusive to her child. Yes, her self and other-directed emotions are also mirrored in her dreams, which, in turn, reflect on the baby's heart. He gets more than a single disappointment or blessing for each feeling-laden thought she has. While in the womb, his facial expressions range from grins to grimaces. Such shows of emotion could come to him from similar ones passed on by mother's (or father's) own feelings and related hormonal changes, no matter if she is awake or dreaming.

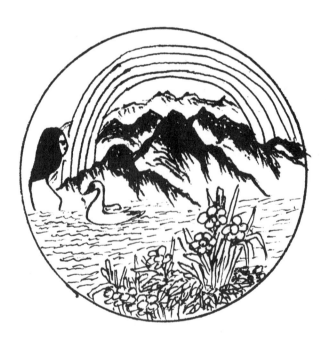

*I dream of a swan, floating by flowers in a lake; it's only you, my child.*

"The interpretation," advises a Korean proverb, "is more important than the dream." Another counsels, "Even a bad dream can be interpreted wisely." This is why a Korean mother tends to interpret her dreams in an affirmative light, and her good intentions undoubtably guide her to a more promising outcome of her dreams. Generally, the dreams are linked to the mother's ever-changing social, physical, and emotional condition, so they vary as the baby develops.

Following the Five Phases approach of the Chinese *Yellow Emperor's Classic of Internal Medicine* as well as folk beliefs as taught to me by elderly Taoist sage Lee Jae Young (in his hilltop tent on the outskirts of Seoul in 1992), I shall offer sample interpretations of dreams collected by university students.

In a conception dream, related by Mrs. Sok, the baby's will to be born won over his mother's initial reluctant heart:

## Eclipse

*I was standing by a house under trees, near a mountain, when a large, red sun approached her. It was smiling. Opening my mouth, I ate it, and so the world became dark. Trying to vomit it out again, I couldn't.*

*I became pregnant but several weeks later began discharging blood, so I went to see a doctor. He told me that I must have an abortion. Instead, I took some herbs. Then the bleeding stopped and I got well. After bearing the baby, a son, I became rich and happy.*

Here the smiling sun was a baby spirit, who gaily entered her womb through the doorway of her mouth. Even though the woman was at first afraid of the mysterious darkness, a possible eclipse of happiness, and wanted to abort it, later she felt compelled, perhaps by the dream baby, to change her mind.

\*　　\*　　\*

A woman might dream of small animals, as did Mrs. Ahn:

# Toads

*I was napping in my small cottage garden, located in a valley surrounded by high mountains, when suddenly several frogs jumped on me and got into my underwear. I was quite surprised. Soon, while I was watching, they began changing into big toads.*

*After ten months, I bore our son. From ancient times, in Korea, a toad has symbolized a son.*

To me, the small frogs changing into larger toads manifest the mother's projected, evolving image of her baby. Entering her underwear signifies conception.

Amphibians also have a "phallic" appearance, indicating a boy. Although this dream might be disturbing to a Westerner and despite the initial surprise and fright, it could be a welcome one, because of the auspicious meaning of a frog to a Korean. In a well-known legend, "Kumwa," a handsome, gold frog = boy was found under a stone by a king and later became his adopted heir.

The assumed "green" frog color, following the Five Phases scheme, relates to the Liver. The behavior of the amphibians suggests an over-active organ and lack of vitality. Generalized fatigue is a sign of conception, so Mrs. Ahn could have taken this as a cue to get sufficient rest.

\*      \*      \*

As the weeks go by, a woman's body heats up in response to feeding the growing life in her womb. She may feel that she is actually "burning up." Mrs. Jo recounts:

# Fire

*Our house was burning up in flames. All the villagers came out of their own houses to watch. They didn't try to put the fire out. I was anxious but they told her, "Don't worry!"*

*Then, snakes curled out of the blaze.*

*Afterwards, my son was born.*

The house could symbolize the (grand)mother's overheating womb. This, rather than an unavoidable fate, is a warning for her to "cool down."

The snakes symbolize her expected child. Fire is an indication of prosperity and also *yang*, active energy, or a male. Looking back, all are favorable signs.

Applying the Five Phases approach, Fire and the color red are also signs of frustrations of the heart. Recognizing this, the dreamer should act to cool down her thoughts. "Don't worry" is apropos.

\* \* \*

Further along, as her womb expands and the woman feels more comfortable with maternity, she may harbor expectations for the success of her child. Mrs. Kim, a housewife, says:

# Salt

*There was a small amount of salt in my house. Then it started increasing and kept on growing until their windows were overflowing.*

*At last, the whole village was filled with salt.*

*I bore a son. He's now a student, majoring in Public Information.*

Again, the house equals the womb. Here, it doesn't suffice to keep the vast amount of wealth (salt = money) she expects to come out of it. Her interest is altruistic, for she wishes to share these riches with the whole village. From this point of view, the dream is auspicious.

Raw salt is blackish: in light of the Five Phases theory, the mother may be experiencing fears, possibly related to over-active kidneys (associated with the color black), which gave rise to her dream. This is further supported by the notion that the flavor associated with the kidneys is salty.

She may, subconsciously, be afraid that her belly is growing so big that it might explode. Being able to bring this fear to the surface of her consciousness could enable her to dismiss it as illusory, on one hand, and, to take steps to bolster her confidence on the other.

*    *    *

The mother is nearing her day of labor, naturally apprehensive of the tell-tale breaking of the water-bag. Mrs. Lee, narrates:

## Flood

*I dreamt of a flood all over the country, but, fortunately, no one was in my house.*

*I climbed up to the top of a mountain and found an apple tree. Although I was delighted to see its small, red apples, the tree was very tall and, eventually, I could reach only one.*

*The apple, my daughter, got rid of my solitude; I felt like the happiest woman in the world.*

Here a cool fear, related to the dark water of the Kidney, changed into a warm joy of the Heart for delivering a fine girl, the red apple. A flood washes away the old life, including the present need for a womb (house) and the mountain represents a new life waiting to be lived on the upside after birth. The fundamental optimism of this dream was something the woman cherished as she neared and began labor. It might even have helped to bring her through.

*   *   *

Next, after the water-bag is broken, a new expectation or apprehension arises: that of the womb gate opening up for giving birth. Mrs. Jung says:

## Dragonquake

*I saw the sky changing to red. Suddenly, thunder rolled and thunderbolts struck the earth. At last, the earth split open, and, from the gap, a gigantic dragon flew high into the sky. A boy was sitting on the dragon's back.*

*The dragon's features were very strange, because it had two heads, yet only one body. Then, as the thunder and lightning was becoming more and more violent, the boy disappeared with the dragon in the sky. At the same time, I woke up.*

Her forward looking dream begins with joy over ensuing labor, followed by the splitting open of her body and the baby bursting out. Whereas a Western woman might have been dismayed at the sight of a two-headed dragon, this beast is an auspicious symbol of fertility and royalty throughout the Far East. In the evolution of a dragon's life, it rises from the motherly sea, or else the bowels of the earth, and ascends to Heaven to become a spiritual king. The boy is, in fact, her child, and he is rising up toward success.

The red sky paints the fire of joy or celebration from the Heart. But too much joy can be exhausting. Of course, by the time of delivery, a mother's natural resources have been fairly well drained, and she will need a full rest for recovery after giving birth.

## Dreaming, "I Love You"

Usually an expectant mother's (or, father's) dreams indicate feelings towards the baby occupying the womb. When she dreams, "I love you…," by grasping a dream flower, for instance, her baby may be gladdened. Mother's breath is melodiously calm and her heart beats out a friendly song. But when she, in a nightmare, dreams, "I hate you…," by fleeing from or hurting a dream animal, for example, he could be saddened and even cry. Mother's breath becomes frenzied, her heart erratic, and he intuits, "because of me…"

He might react physically, gripping his tiny fists and feet in his own dream; for during a good portion of his time in the womb, a baby dreams. Or, if awake, he could pound on the curve of Mother's womb with his fists or kick at it, too. With a mix of signals from both body and heart, he fathoms how she feels about him and responds accordingly.

Almost every mother (and father) has hostile feelings, periodically, in dreams; for example, after she falls asleep upset and exhausted from a noisy, confusing day. But these feelings can be easily offset by other, naturally tender, caring emotions which she may offer her babe. Airing feelings such as "Precious child, I'm always with you" could be comforting.

## Incubating a Dream

*Relax from head to toe, while breathing calmly, lovingly, from the womb.*

*See an adorable baby dancing, affectionately pinching your ear.*

*Kiss its cheeks and caress its body with a genuine feeling of care.*

*Whisper, while drifting off to sleep, "I'm going to visit you in my dreams tonight!"*

# Conversing with a Friend

"A pregnant queen in China was obliged to address the baby in her womb with a respectful, 'O King,' if the court physicians or diviners had concluded that it would be a first-born male," says our Chinese guest, Mrs. Wang Su Yi. "She would politely ask questions, such as, 'O King, is there anything you would like me to do?' 'O King, would you care for an apple?' 'O King, is this music to your liking?' 'O King, shall we go for a stroll in the garden?'"

"O Queen," Young Im offers, "would you care for a cup of citron tea?"

Oh Song Hee, a high school teacher in Seoul, agrees with age-old beliefs, explaining,

> I'm sure our baby could hear me when she was inside my wife's belly.
>
> Sometimes my wife would complain, 'Honey, the baby's kicking my belly and moving all about. I feel so helpless; what can I do!?' Whenever she would speak in such a way, I would lay my head on her belly and try to persuade the baby, saying, 'Come on, Baby. You should be good and generous. I'm sure you're a good baby.' Occasionally, I would talk to her about some professional tennis players, including Steffi Graff and Boris Becker.
>
> She's now just sixteen months old. She's very active, behaves like a boy, and is quite strong. She has a beautiful smile and likes to smile very much. I think this is because during my wife's pregnancy, I used to lay my head on her belly and say, 'Smile, Baby; smiling makes you happy and beautiful.'
>
> Also, during pregnancy, my wife regularly played an English language tape. I'm not sure, but now, maybe because of that, my daughter seems to understand when I speak to her in English.

Mr. Oh intuited how to draw close to his evolving child and give her encouragement. Your spouse can do so, too, by laying his ear lightly on the bulge of your belly and listening quietly to the movements of the reality of life within. This is something you can't do.[14] Once your spouse becomes aware of the baby, which indeed is a startling discovery, with his cheek against your flesh, he can start talking affectionately to her and perhaps puckering his lips up close for a kiss. The heart and lips of your man will be near your child's attentive ear, so they can get better acquainted through such exchanges day by day. She might even try to kiss him back!

My Yugoslavian colleague, Jovan Deretic, Ph.D., concurs: "Once, while my wife was pregnant with our daughter, she got very scared and told me, 'The baby hasn't moved for some days. I'm worried that something awful's happened to it!'

"So I placed my ear on her belly and listened. The moment my ear touched my wife's skin, the baby kicked the very same place, surprising me. Our daughter has a good sense of humor; that was her first joke!"

They must have laughed quite a bit after that, though a pregnant woman should laugh with moderation, not to frighten the child. If the parents display a sense of humor during pregnancy, smiling over the surprises and ironies of life, all the more chance of their baby having one, too.

In 1993, during the seventh month of my wife's pregnancy with our second daughter, Young Im says, "Feel this ... No, more over on the left side; when I turn over, it goes, 'Bluck, bluck...'"

I reply, "It's bobbing up again against my hand; I can feel it very clearly.

'Little one, we're waiting for you. Your mother and I care for you...'"

While I am talking, there is no motion below my hand, but when I finish, the child moves on like a gentle wave.

Yoo An Jin, Ph.D., a professor of Child Psychology at Seoul National University describes how a traditional woman believed that her baby could hear and understand her words from early in pregnancy.

She would speak to it. As it grew older and seemed to be responding with various movements, kicks, and punches, she would say, 'My baby wants to learn some more words.'

Or she might say, 'My baby's talking to me!'

## A Fancied Conversation

*"How are you, darling …? O.K. …? I'm feeling so delightfully lazy, like a mother cat … Yawning, and stretching carefully …*

*"Oh, you poked me … Of course, it doesn't hurt … Yes, I adore you …*

*"Now, I'm opening the curtain … The sun's rising; can you see the light? It's glowing on the plum blossoms …*

*"Can you feel its rays? Soft and warm on my skin …"*

## Reading to a Budding Scholar

*A king climbs a mountain to his ancestral shrine. He bows, offers rice and wine, then prays, "How can I find good men to help me govern my country?"*

*A booming voice from above says, "They must receive a good education concerning the relationship of Heaven and Earth."*

*The king asks, "But, when is the best time for their education to begin?"*

*"Of course, while they're still in the womb!"*

Yasumi Inose, a Japanese NHK T.V. documentary director, informs us that,

> Teaching to the womb was practiced by (aristocratic) parents in Imperial China to give their babies an early start for the highly competitive, civil service examinations.
>
> These exams were required for many important public positions. Out of thousands of applicants, only a small percentage passed (the usual, four-day tests). That's why most parents would begin preparing a child as early as possible.

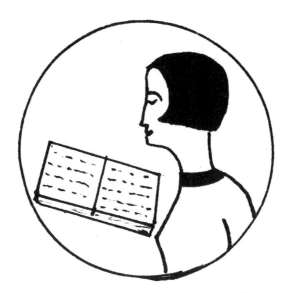

*Let's read only words of beauty and wisdom.*

Since a baby in the womb was believed to absorb its mother's passion for study, a pregnant woman was asked to memorize and recite proverbs drawn from classics, including *The Book of Odes*, *The Analects of Confucius*, *The Doctrine of the Golden Mean*, and *The Works of Mencius*.

"When an expectant mother woke up in the morning," states Liu Jia He, a professor of History at Beijing Normal University, "she looked at the wall and read a strip of calligraphy holding a fitting proverb for her baby."

Such expressions of wisdom and beauty were offered "in a very loud voice to the baby in the womb," says Chinese mother Wang Su Yi.

\*　　\*　　\*

In 1336, Lee Pyon Hanguk Pae Puin *(Great Korean Wife)* discovered her conception after an unusual dream (recorded in Lee Bong Ju's, *Story of Chong Mong Ju*):

She wakes up trembling, then shakes her husband.
　　"What's the matter?"
　　"I just dreamt a frightening dream."

"What was it? Tell me quickly!"

"I was carrying a flowerpot full of orchids in my hands, then accidently dropped it on the ground. The pot shattered, but the orchids were unharmed."

After she blurts out her dream, he bursts out laughing.

"Why are you laughing!"

"That was a *Tae Mong* (Fetus Dream). You're going to have a baby!"

"But, what about the broken flowerpot!?"

"That's a good sign, too. Though the pot was broken, the orchids were unharmed. An orchid's a symbol for a virtuous scholar. We'll surely have a scholarly son."

Much impressed by her husband's words, she sets about guiding the child in her womb. She decides, *"I will make the best son of all time!"* Besides the traditional forms of *Embryonic Education*, she gives great emphasis to her own learning.

She asserts, "Women have to strive during pregnancy to follow the ways of previous wise mothers, reading books about them and affirming to themselves, *'I want to have a son just like hers!'*"

Also, Mrs. Lee strives to practice justice in everything she does, hoping to instill in her child a sense of fairness.

Just prior to giving birth, she dreams that a dragon flies down, filling up her bedroom.

As a result of her efforts, in 1337, she bore an exceptional son, Chong Mong (Dragon Dream) Ju. He grew up to become an eminent Confucian poet and scholar, as well as a government minister, who carried much sway in the court of the last Wang dynasty ruler of the Koryo kingdom (918–1392). However, Chong Mong died from an usurper's blow, out of loyalty to his beleaguered king, his head cracked open like the pot of orchids.

\*     \*     \*

During the Choson Dynasty (1392–1910) in Korea, the teaching of Confucian classics also began in the womb, with hopes that the baby would acquire the attributes of a sage.

Lee Won Sup writes in The Royal Family's Teaching for Raising Life (1993) "From six months of pregnancy, a eunuch would go to the queen's court and read. In the evening, a court girl would continue reading. The books, all recited in a beautiful voice, included the classic *One Thousand* Chinese Characters, Etiquette, and *Proverbs*."

"While sitting in front of the pregnant queen, the servants were requested to, 'Always use a loud voice, with beautiful pronunciation, reading clearly; hold a white jade stick for pointing at the letters; read variously, with a high or low sound, and a long or short rhythm; move your body right and left in a regular rhythm to remember sentences.' Variation stimulates and sends meaning to the brain."

"Our ancestors felt that a mother's behavior influenced her baby," reports Mr. Yoo, a college student. "Therefore, they preferred a pregnant woman to be as diligent, patient, and polite as possible. Like other mothers, my grandmother had to get up at 5 A.M. to express her respect for her elders, and especially to read a lot of good books, because my great-grandfather (he was a king in our family then) hoped that her coming baby would become a writer or a teacher. She sometimes says that she read 'almost a thousand books' during pregnancy. She truly believes that it swayed my father to become an ardent reader and a wonderful teacher."

Choice reading (for example, the *I-Ching*, written by Queen Jin's son, King Wen) is a means of broadening one's horizons and cultivating one's own virtues, as well as passing them on to the child in the womb. The finer the quality of readings (such as poetry, nature philosophy, and folk tales) you offer yourself and your child, the deeper your souls can grow, and the more comfortable you will feel living in this increasingly close family of our planet Earth.

\*     \*     \*

For another inspiring dream of conception, Miss Sok, a student, reports:

*In the midst of lightning flashes, two hermits appeared before my mother. They showed her two books, one empty and the other filled with words, and said, "Choose one."*

*So she chose the one with words.*

The dream means that I'll be a great scholar.

## Seeing the World from a Star

Mr. Joh, a university student, claims,"I became a Christian while in my mother's womb, because she attended church regularly while she was pregnant."

"In former days," Sung Oo, a Buddhist monk, states in his book, *T'ae Gyo 'Embryonic Education'* (1986), "a blind person would be invited into a home to recite the *Diamond Sutra* before a woman with child." This gave mother and child spiritual protection and a feeling for the faith.

Lee Won Sup, in his *Royal Family's Teaching for Raising Life* (1996) adds, "In the royal courts of Tang in China, Buddhist holy texts were recited in a splendid voice by a eunuch for the queen from five months of pregnancy to make her peaceful."

To ensure that the child grows up without prejudice, the parents could occasionally page though "sacred books" of faiths other than those of their own. They could recognize that there are countless spiritual paths claiming to be "the only one," and that a good many of them are actually vari-colored leaves on the same divine tree. Each parent could open a compassionate, glowing heart, spreading branches of tranquility and love over the world.

## Merits of Love

A baby's heart is originally full of light and open-ended, has space for and, for all we know, may already contain, the whole Universe.

Whether African or American, Asian or European, from conception, the baby has a chance to bring more harmony to this world by feeling in the womb our shared humanity and intermingled fate, and how, despite diverse customs, to love our neighbors.

As you grow more clear and tender, the atmosphere of your heart changes. It becomes finer, clearer, free of habitual thinking. This reassuring air drifts down to your attending child.

She or he feels in the womb, more than at any other time of her life, the glow of a secret grace that is beyond all creeds and illumines our hearts.

## Grandmother's Last Words

*Grandmother smiled ....*

*Already her face was wrinkled and pocked, like a kindly, old moon's. "Marry a rainbow girl, free of all stain of nations, colors, and religions; she, being one and all."*

*Strangely, I remember how Grandma touched the back of my hand with her dry, soft fingers, and at the same time pushed a plateful of warm, freshly-baked cookies and a glass of milk at me as if I were a child. Upon reflection, I was, and still am ....*

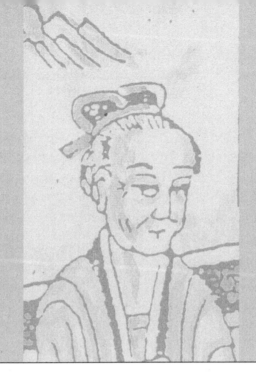

# Delivering Your Baby

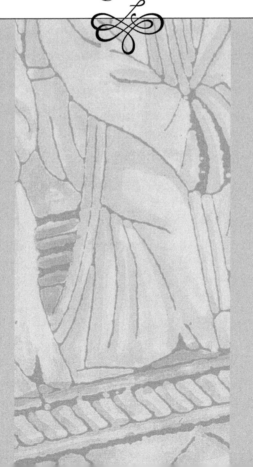

*I see a beautiful baby on the other side of a footbridge, which arches over a pond filled with lilies, and, in the waters below, many gods and goddesses are bathing.*

*It is a boy and his arms are reaching out for me. I cross over the bridge and pick him up.*

—a Nepalese woman's dream

\*     \*     \*

*I am climbing a hill on a moonlit night when I hear the sounds of people singing, celebrating. Creeping up behind a tree, I see twelve gods wearing animal masks, dancing in a circle around a jolly baby boy. They play all night, much to the joy of the laughing baby.*

*As dawn breaks, the gods disappear, and the baby is left alone, smiling up at me. As he is a boy, I creep over and gather him up in my arms.*

—a Korean woman's dream

*Prissy is carrying me through a woods on her ample shoulders, but when I venture to suggest, "Be careful…," leaves and branches brushing up against my face, she sings out in those wondrous tones of hers, "Just keep the faith…!"*

*We meet a forlorn Ethiopian woman on the path by a hut, and Prissy tosses a cotton doll down to her. Smiling up, she says, "I've never seen anyone as fine as you!"*

—the author's dream

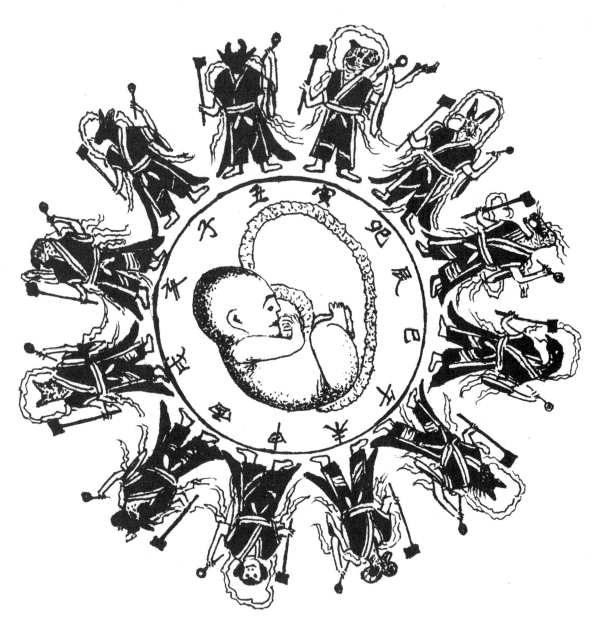

*You sleep in the universe of my womb, protected by the twelve animal gods of the Zodiac.*

# On the Way to a Birth

One fall morning, descending along an alley in Seoul with my Indian friend Sheikh Mohammed Iqbal, I notice a young pregnant mother, accompanied by an older woman, perhaps her mother-in-law, walking across from us. The gravid one is tall, in a loose, off-white dress, but her normally handsome facial features appear sickly and tightly drawn. Her belly is protruding out of her comely body like a honeydew melon.

Fortunately, I have my camera, for I desire to take her picture for our *Hand Book* but am embarrassed to ask. What if I, an unkempt foreigner, surprise her by my request, and her baby, then, "pops out?"

But my attention is diverted by Iqbal, who is remarking on the stunning string of burgundy morning glories trailing off the cement wall on our side of the street. Then he holds out a vineful in his delicate brown hand for me to photograph.

Meanwhile, the women have wobbled by us along the opposite wall, heading for an underpass. Suddenly, the ailing woman leans against the wall, grasping her belly in pain, while her companion, maybe her mother-in-law, stands passively beside her. She's been through all this, at least once, herself.

The idea astounds me. She's having labor pains! She's on the way to a birth! The baby will be born, perhaps any minute!

I desire this picture, but there is no way. The pregnant one's lovely raven hair is trailing against the high, sloping concrete wall, much like one of the open morning glories on the other side where we stand.

I cannot, in decency, linger any longer, ogling her unsteady progress of a few yards at a time, clutching herself in pain, her fair head against the wall. So we proceed under the tunnel, which is painted with yellow and black tigress stripes on either end.

We are well ahead as they emerge on the far side, making their agonizing way a few yards at a time, still sixty or so yards away from the local women's clinic.

Only when we get farther on do I dare point my lens and get a secret shot of the woman facing us—enduring labor contractions, carrying her own self and her baby's on their way to the birth.

# Beautiful Bodies

*Shut your eyes, or leave them partially open. Mentally journey through the body, from head to toes, attending to and loving it part by part. Say, "Relax this young and beautiful body."*

*Peer through the mind's eye into the pink, circular chasm of the earth's womb beneath your feet, sensing the hollows there.*

*Inhale and gently say, "F-E-R-T-I-L-I-T-Y."*

*Imagine the fog of life wisping up from pink flowering vines to the toes, then, around your ankles and knees.*

*Draw it along your thighs and on through into the womb.*

*Feel its sensation spiraling about an affectionate baby, who is joined by a stalk to a fresh sunflower, which brightens up the womb.*

*When exhaling, disseminate "F-E-R-T-I-L-I-T-Y" over the rest of your body.*

*Gaze at an orange gem in your navel, and recall the looping stem of a flower that connected it in the womb to your own mother. Behind this, your own baby is waiting; his (or her) small inner light flickering through the pores.*

*Reflect on the sound and sensation of "G-R-E-A-T H-O-P-E-S" in the womb. See each letter written in orange-gold glitter. After a few moments, combine these into one glittering sun, which circulates around your body.*

## Going Around in Buddha's Womb

In the winter of 1989, as we climb by curling rows of candle-lit lamps into the sanctuary of a Buddhist temple near Osaka, Japan, night falls. It is cold inside.

My companion, Yasumi Inose, leads the way down a short, wooden staircase, brushing through a slit in long, black draperies.

Suddenly it is pitch-dark; I don't know where we are, or why we have journeyed underground. I can't feel the walls on either side and mumble nervously, "Do you mind if I hold on to your shoulder?"

Yasumi doesn't and, comforted, I creep with him through utter darkness, turning now and again, while the entire chamber echoes with a chorus of chanting.

At one spot, the chanting is just above us. Then, turning a corner, a bit of light shines through. An altar is in an alcove with three tiny, gold Buddhas seated in meditation. I bow respectfully, and soon again we are in utter darkness. Cautiously, we shuffle on and on, the chanting resounding in our ears.

Yasumi says, "I found it! I found the lock! Here, turn it. It's for good luck."

After fumbling about, I feel the cold handle of a bar lock, and squeak it (symbolizing some sort of opening up) to and fro. (Unfortunately, I get my finger stuck and only with effort can pull it out!).

All is pitch dark again. Then, around a bend, more draperies brush my head as we emerge at the foot of another flight of stairs.

Yasumi elucidates, "It is called the *'T'ai Nai Meguri.'* Or, 'Going Around in Buddha's Womb.' Women who wish to conceive a baby and already pregnant ones, too, go in there to get purified so that their babies will be born with good fortune." Upon hearing that, I decide to climb back down again; this time alone.

Leaving my guide, I grope through the circular womb of Buddha, thrice more, now aware of the birth canal walls on either side. I strive to die in the darkness and be born over and over again, the song of Buddha ringing through my body and spirit. But the effect does not really strike me until the third pilgrimage, when I notice a young couple, with the woman carrying an infant in her arms, walking ahead of me. Of course, I can't see them, and the baby is silent, at first. Slowly, it begins to whimper and, once in a while, let out a cry. The woman's voice reassures it. It is quiet, tentatively whimpers, then cries out again. *Now, I feel like I'm really in a womb!*

## Visions of Birth

*Close your eyes. Breathe in the gift of life, and let it out into a grove of cypress trees.*

*See yourself promenading around a pond of white lotuses.*

*Go up to a wavy tree, and gracefully grasp a fragrant, pink flowering branch.*

*Stretch out gently, as the golden breath of life surges through your limbs.*

*Cry out joyfully, as your child emerges and is born.*

## Our Daughter's Birth

One winter's day in 1982, I pray earnestly to the Spirit of the Universe "for a close and loving friend," yes, "a daughter," before our union....

Young Im dreams that a small snake wriggles across the floor and bites her forearm. She wakes up and exclaims, "Oh, a snake bit me! I have to tell my mother!"

More than nine months pass, then, one evening, she begins feeling mild contractions in her uterus, which continue on through the night. At about 4 A.M., she calls tremulously from the couch, where she lays curled up in a ball, "Jeremy, I think it's time for us to go to the hospital!"

A few minutes later, I return with the taxi, which carries us to the nearby Seoul Seventh Day Adventist Hospital.

After we step into the waiting room, a doctor, dressed in green operating clothes, glances at my wife's dress and says, "Ma'am, your belly's very large. You'll probably need a Caesarian.…"

Soon, we are fleeing the scary hospital; a cold-hearted Caesarian operation is the last thing we wanted! Thank goodness, we had already made alternative arrangements with an experienced mid-wife. Young Im is clutching her belly in pain. I hail a taxi and we speed over hills to the midwife's house, about fifteen minutes away.

Getting there, the midwife feels my wife's quivering belly and examines her dilating cervix. "You've arrived just in time. Step over into the delivery room, quickly!" she says.

Young Im stretches out upon a simple rubber mat on the floor. Then the midwife and her grown daughter begin coaching our baby out, while I kneel by Young Im's side. "Push woman, push!," the midwife urges, but my wife's face becomes apple red and her eyes bloodshot with strain.

"Just a moment, wait," I say, gesturing to all with my hands. "Sweetie, push with your belly, not with your eyes." And I dab some persimmon-leaf tea on her dry lips with a handkerchief.

The midwife and her daughter coach her again, "Push woman, push!" Yet, despite several minutes of Young Im's struggling, our baby won't come out. Maybe something is wrong.…

"Wait; rest a moment, darling," I say, spreading my hands to signal the mid-wives to stop. They pause reluctantly. Soon, after Young Im catches her breath, I tell them, "O.K., let's try again, now.…"

The midwife and her daughter appeal to her, "Push woman, push hard! Hard!" Young Im tries for several minutes more, to no avail.

Finally, I shout, "Wait…!" It occurs to me that the baby might be hesitating to come out amidst so much excitement, and that if my wife would simply relax a bit that could encourage them both.

Bewildered, the midwife and her daughter gape as I lean over to press acupressure points on the inner sides of Young Im's calves *(Three Yin Meeting)* with my thumbs, and, after a few moments, on others *(Four Doors)* between the webs of her big toes *(Big Joining)* and the webs of her thumbs *(Uniting Valley)*. While gradually pressing them with increasing intensity, I say, "Now, once more…."

The midwife urges, "Push woman, push!" Soon a bloody, gelatinous mass appears at the gate of the womb. "Oh no," I think, "its head's all mashed up!"

"Push woman, push more…!," the midwife and her daughter persist. At last, a full head appears and the baby slides out by itself. It starts choking. The midwife uses a tube to suction liquid out of its mouth. Then, the baby cries. Still bloody, it is placed on Young Im's nipple, a surprisingly thick umbilical cord coiling behind.

I've seen its face; all wrinkly and old. It looks just like my grandfather—but he is long gone.

And this baby is—"A girl!" We are glad and hug her. Later, we name her "Chalina," after my grandfather, Charles. "Charlina" would have been too hard sounding a name for a girl, but "Cha" means "Tea" in Korean and "lina" could be "Lena" the Swan.

Near dawn, we are reclining in the delivery room on quilted mattresses, our daughter between us. While Young Im sleeps, I set a hand on Chalina's tiny, sleeping chest. Suddenly, a gentle, warm current creeps into my hand and rises up my arm into my heart, filling it with what I fancy to be our daughter's spirit; she must recognize how I've been waiting for her. She already is a close, loving friend.

## Angelic Child

*Close your eyes lightly. Say, "B-L-O-S-S-O-M-I-N-G," as you and baby drift off in a boat around a lily-spotted lake, followed by curious swans, who circle 'round and 'round.*

*See a glittering emerald (or a pink crystal) by your heart. Say, and feel, "T-E-N-D-E-R-N-E-S-S," while nursing a small boy or girl at your breast.*

*Imagine the angelic child growing up: one, two, three months.... S(he) clasps your fingers, toddling along a soft, sandy shore by your side.*

## All's Well in the Baby's Universe

After returning home with our newly born daughter, Young Im chooses to stay indoors to help her through a fragile initiation into the world. She won't venture out into the daylight for the customary one hundred days (other women offer a minimum of twenty-one days) of post-natal care. This is called *Sanhu (Following delivery) Jori (Caring for a body and mind that has become weak so as to restore it to health).*

Young Im is careful when she lays the child's head and body on the quilt, shifting it from time to time, shaping it evenly on the back and sides.

Resting, she takes only moderate exercise. She eats warm, nourishing food, particularly seaweed soup, to cleanse her body and improve circulation (whale and dolphin cows consume seaweed after delivery, too) as well as carp soup, for enhancing breast milk. For three days after birth, until her milk is flowing, she offers Chalina only drops of colostrum. Nature provides the baby stored-up nutrition during that time, while clearing the black feces from her intestines.

Going out into a busy life too soon, exposing herself to drafts and damp weather, drinking chilled juice, or taking cold showers could weaken my wife's body, reducing the chances of a full recovery. She has gone through a serious ordeal. She must relax mentally and physically, avoiding extremes of temperature and emotions. Nature needs time to mend a womb, replenish the body, and prepare it for a new life style. She says, "It takes one hundred days for a woman's bones to regain their normal position after giving birth."

Otherwise, as was the experience of one of our neighbors, she might suffer from chronic aches and pains all over the body and not wholly recover from the ordeal of pregnancy, save by getting pregnant again and being more careful then. Remaining at home also helps increase bonds with the baby, who is "handled with her whole heart," while the immune system strengthens and protects her against "impure" presences. Old books caution that these could be acquaintances emitting the stenches of tobacco, wine, or erotic yearnings; gossipy or jealous neighbors (with "an evil eye"); persons with contagious diseases or mental disorders; ones whose families have recently been visited by death; those who have just returned from adventurous, far journeys; and other such questionable cases. Young Im knows from old stories how fragile an infant can be, open to all influences, negative and positive, so she doesn't take any chances.

A heart-felt spirit, her own mother is also there to help out. To warn others against violating our sacred space, she stretches a straw, braided rope, laced with pine needles (to ward off ghosts), red peppers (symbol of a boy), and sticks of charcoal (symbol of a girl) over our doorway. Only family members and close relatives can pass under.

As for them, our little child is theirs, too. Theirs to cuddle, to adore and, above all, through their own faithful, considerate behavior, to guide towards a virtuous life.

During those one hundred days, the guidance given our baby before birth continues outside the womb. The playing of soft, spirited music, the viewing of colorful paintings, the reading aloud of poems, the constant flow of tender conversation between mother, father, and child, the caresses, the nutritious diet, and so forth, all continue through a debut into the sunny outdoors of birds, flowers, and butterflies, other gleeful children, and affectionate, inquiring friends.

\*     \*     \*

Six weeks pass: Young Im, your honey milk suits our baby perfectly. She is touching your nipples, clinging to you, carried blissfully about all day, never losing contact with your flesh, often gazing in your eyes.

During the night, she sleeps between us. We are like one body and mind. She'll be more confident in later years for it and honor you for your gracious sacrifices; you, too, will care for her more. She'll feel more at ease, touching and helping others in her turn, too.

You carry her in your arms or on your back, wrapped up in a five-colored, silk, tie-around blanket, her ear attending to the reassuring beat of your heart. Tranquil, she rides and dances high above the ground, hardly ever crying, for she feels safe, at home.

# Sarasvati's Milk

It is the winter of 1989. I've been a guest for a week at Saikoji, an isolated Buddhist monastery tucked away in a hilly forest near Kyoto, Japan. As I depart, the monks lead me to an orange doll-house shrine by an icy creek and begin chanting prayers for a safe journey.

"Jeremy, come on down and try the milk of the goddess!" the old Zen master calls up. I leap off the bank beside the creek's fresh flowing water and cross over slippery stones to the other side.

"This is the milk of Sarasvati (Indian goddess of Music and Learning)," he says, as I lift my lips to receive an arc of sweet water surging through the hollow of one of her stone breasts. It is icy and delicious. I drink from it and from her other breast for a while until the monks call me away. I feel as if I have been recovering my own lost mother and then realize that the water was a gift of generosity and life I can share with mothers and fathers from all over the world through this guide.

"Two hundred or so years ago," the old monk continues, "one of the Emperor's wives could not produce enough milk for her child, so she came to this shrine and drank from the breasts of the beautiful goddess, Sarasvati. Now women journey here, even from far away, when they have difficulty producing milk. They pray to Sarasvati and drink from her breasts. Afterwards, their own milk begins to flow."

## A Fountain of Love

*Silently say, "S-W-E-E-T J-O-Y," feel a blue fountain bubbling from one's chest, up to the lips. Eyes glisten merrily.*

## Water Babies

In the winter of 1989, on an early morning walk in Osaka, Japan, I come upon an area of secluded Buddhist temples. Around gardens and courtyards I wander and everywhere am struck by the recurrence of small, child-like statues, many with red or white bibs around their necks and some wearing caps. I ask my companion, Yasumi Inose, "What are these for?"

"They're for '*Mizukos*,' 'Water babies.' Miscarried, or aborted children."

"Are there so many abortions in Japan?"

"Yes, these days and before, too. Now the Mizukos are often the children of unfortunate love affairs. After the war, almost every family had someone who'd aborted a child, out of poverty."

I reflect that I, too, was born soon after World War II ended. If I had been of Japanese parents, then I might have been aborted, too. "But, why the statues?"

"The statues are *Jizos*, little Buddhas, donated by the mothers of *Mizukos*. They pray that their baby will journey on to be born again as a Buddha. They think that if they don't do this, the dead baby will come back to haunt them. Every misfortune that might befall them would be attributed to its' vengeful spirit. Furthermore, if they don't pray, their baby could carry on their bad karma and have an unfortunate love life in its next existence, too. The mothers feel very guilty over losing a child. That's why they pray, really: to try to free themselves from the guilt."

If by misfortune you should lose your baby, you could shape a clay statuette of it. Paint in eyes and mouth, then set it on your mantelpiece. Give it a smile of contentment. Pray deep in your heart for the safe and loving passage of its soul.

## Mother Peace Credo

1) I've been blessed by a baby.

2) I'm in love with him (her).

3) I'm living for our happiness.

4) I'm smiling at our neighbors.

5) I'm seeing beauty everywhere.

6) I'm finding goodness in everyone.

7) I'm forgiving others' follies.

8) I'm sharing joy with everything.

9) I'm offering peace to our planet.

10) I'm showing our children how to love.

# Appendices

## An Ancient Pregnancy Moon Calender

About 1,500 years ago in the Northern Chi kingdom, Dr. Hsu Chi Tsai devoted much care to the needs of pregnant women and their babies. In Taichung, during the summer of 1990, I found that his *Golden Principle* is still being studied by students at Taiwan's prestigious China Medical College. In his book, Dr. Hsu offers this lunar calender program for pregnancy:

**1st (lunar) Month:** The food you eat should be well-cooked and refined. Soup ought to be on the sour side. You should eat a lot of barley and wheat, but shun spicy food, or meat with a strong smell, like lamb.

The Yin (female) pulse is lacking, so don't use acupuncture (at specific points). The blood circulation is not smooth, so don't work hard. Sleep in a quiet area to avoid disturbances and fear.

**2nd Month:** You should not eat spicy food, or the internal organs of animals. Stay in a tranquil place and don't receive any acupuncture.

**3rd month:** If you want to bear a son, play with a bow and arrow. If you wish for a girl, toy with a pearl necklace or other ornaments.

Avoid being sad, overly worried, or frightened. Your palm is related to your pulse, so don't get acupuncture there.

**4th Month:** Eat more rice and fish, goose or duck soup. These help the blood circulate, but don't eat too much.

**5th Month:** Sleep longer and get up late. After taking a bath, put on thick clothes immediately. Always keep warm and avoid cold air and cold places.

Eat rice and wheat flour. Beef and mutton are now good; for this month the mother needs to cultivate her *ch'i*, which flows through a cycle of twelve vessels in her body). Don't undereat, overeat, get hot, dry, or too tired.

**6th Month:** You can do some physical exercise. Go out for a stroll. Watch a dog or horse run. Eat the flesh of ferocious wild animals, like an eagle or a tiger. These can help strengthen your back and nerves. But, even if it is tasty, don't eat too much.

**7th Month:** You can do some physical exercise. Go out for a stroll so that the blood and *ch'i* in your body circulate together. Your bodily movements will also toughen your bones. Don't speak loudly or cry out.

Your residence should be dry. Stay out of very cold air. Don't wear thin clothes, bathe, or eat cold food. Eat rice. Chew often to strengthen your teeth. Your baby's skin and hair have already been formed.

**8th Month:** You should sit peacefully and rest quietly. Don't use too much energy. Avoid eating dry food and irregular meals. Don't hold bowel movements.

**9th Month:** Your baby is already formed. Eat some sweet foods. Your movements should be smooth and slow to protect your baby. Don't stay in a wet or cold area or overdress.

**10th Month:** The five major organs and six corresponding hollow receptacles of the body have been fully developed. Now the *ch'i* can flow through freely. The *ch'i* of Heaven and earth is already concentrated in the baby's *Tan T'ien* (an inch below its navel), therefore the spirit and energy vessels in all its major limbs are already fully developed. The time has come to wait for the baby to be born.

# Modern Acupuncture For Pregnancy

During the summer of 1990, Julia J. Tsuei M.D., a celebrated, Western-trained gynecologist, gave a talk at the China Medical College in Taichung, Taiwan, where I was taking an acupuncture class. She described her experiences in mainland China, and at the Foundation for East-West Medicine in Hawaii, as she was gradually discovering the benefits of acupuncture for pregnant women:

Acupuncture needles are inserted by doctors to regulate the flow of *ch'i* in a person's body by either stimulating or sedating it. Among other uses, they can improve an expectant mother's ability to absorb nutrients from food, normalize her weight, ease the pain of her labor and facilitate the delivery of her child.

To satisfy the curiosity of Western doctors and lay persons, I am including a few details of treatment here.

**Appetite:** Points Stomach 36 (Tsu San Li) on each side of the stomach meridian (bio-energetic channel) may be needled to aid a pregnant woman's digestion. (For safety's sake, follow up with mild heating of dried mugwort (moxibustion) on certain points, including Stomach 36, since it not only stimulates appetite and improves absorption of food but also strengthens the body against miscarriage.)

**Preventing Premature Birth:** Dr. Tsuei says, "Out of twelve habitual aborters in Hawaii, only one did not carry to term after being needled at Spleen 4 (Kuing Sun) on both sides of the spleen meridian twice a week until delivery. This point activates the sensory part of the autonomic nervous system."

**Turning Breech:** While in mainland China, Dr. Tsuei learned that laser acupuncture on point Bladder 67 (Chih Yin) of the bladder meridian was used successfully in 79% of 119 cases for turning a baby around to a proper position in the womb, usually between 30 and 40 weeks of pregnancy. When back in Hawaii, she gave a mild needle stimulation to a friend whose baby was in a breech position, and the next day "the baby was kicking and moving strongly about"—it had turned from its uncomfortable position and was more free.

**Inducing Labor:** When points Liver 4 (Chung Feng) of the liver meridian and Spleen 6 (San Yin Chuan) of the spleen meridian (the most important point for treating women's ailments) were needled on both sides of women in Hawaii, Dr. Tsuei observed contractions beginning twelve and a half minutes later.

**Reducing Contractions and Pain:** Points Spleen 3 (Tai Pai) on both sides of the spleen meridian were helpful where the labor pains become too prolonged and severe to bear, and the mother needed a respite.

**Recalling Contractions:** By needling Liver 3 (Tai Chung) regular contractions came back, without pain.

**Anesthesia:** When desiring to numb the perineum (between the anus and sexual organs), to avoid the pain of possible tearing at delivery or of stitches afterwards, points Liver 4, Stomach 36 and Spleen 6 were needled. In China, ear acupuncture on Shenmen (God's Gate) and the Uterine point were used.

\*    \*    \*

"Acupuncture is a very safe technique," Dr. Tsuei claims, "Its effects apply only where a problem occurs. When the baby is mature, acupuncture will assist in delivery; if not, it won't work."

However, she cautions, "If a person is already feeling pain and is nervous when you start to use needles, they won't work. In such a circumstance, stop contractions with Spleen 4 (Kuing Sun). This will calm the patient down so she will trust you. Then, insert needles in Spleen 6 and Liver 3 to renew the contractions."

If electro-acupuncture is employed for anesthesia, points should be linked by the wires on only one side of the body, so the current does not cross over the heart or womb. Also, only mild stimulation should be given at a frequency below 10 Hertz.

**Post-C-section Pain:** In case of a Caesarian-section, points Liver 4 and Spleen 6 can serve to reduce pain after the operation.

Of course it is not necessary for a layman to follow these details, but I hope a sense of the possibilities of acupuncture in reducing the travails of a woman during pregnancy and delivery can be acquired from the above information.

Still, aside from these specifics, it is best to avoid using acupuncture (as well as moxibustion) because, as Korean acupuncturist, Han Yoon Gi succinctly puts it, "Whenever you give acupuncture to the mother, you are also giving it to her baby."

As more women inquire of the medical community about Chinese-style therapy, the more likely corresponding services will appear in the West. For more information or professional assistance, Dr. Tsui's clinic is listed in the Honolulu phone directory.

# Notes

1.  This body of research has been gathered in a double issue of the *Journal of Prenatal and Perinatal Psychology and Health*, Vol.14:1 and 2, 1999. It can be ordered from apppah@aol.com.

2.  Translated by James Legge.

3.  Adapted from Chin Fuzheng's, *A Collection of Pediatrics* (1750).

4.  This Chinese character (心) is shaped like a physical heart. The heart is considered to be the seat of the spirit, or the force of consciousness, personality, and thoughts.

5.  Translated by Ilza Veith.

6.  Translated by James Legge.

7.  In Legge's notes to *The Book of Odes*.

8.  Adapted from Im Dong Ku's *T'ae* (1970).

9.  *Korea Times*, August 7, 1999.

10. *Ibid*.

11. Translated by James Legge.

12. Designed by Mr. Ahn Jae Sun.

13. *T'ae Gyo Umak* (Embryonic Education Music) Seoul Audio Inc., 1997.

14. Unless with the portable *Hi Bebe!* communicator, produced in 2000 by the S.K. Group of Korea. Among other dialogue features, contains a microphone for the mother; and a feeler with which she can browse over her belly in order to hear the unborn baby's heartbeat, sounds of hiccups, leg kicks, and other movements. However, with any form of artificial device, including music and language tapes, one should act in moderation.

# Sources

An Jin Yoo. *Child-rearing in Traditional Korean Society.* Seoul: Jeongmin Sa, 1982.

_____. *Traditional Korean Society's Early Childhood Education.* Seoul: Seoul University Press, 1990.

Byoung Key Song. (ed.) *Textbook of Oriental Gynecology.* Seoul: Ham Lim, 1978.

Chamberlain, David. *The Mind of Your Newborn Baby.* Berkeley, CA: North Atlantic Books, 1998.

Che Sam Sup and Pak Chon Guk. *A New Theory for an Embryo's Education.* Seoul: Song Bo Sa, 1992.

Fuzheng Chin. *A Collection of Pediatrics.* Beijing: Ching Dynasty, 1750.

Haw Jun. *The Eastern Medical Treasure.* Seoul: 1610.

Im Dong Ku. *T'ae.* Seoul: Oo Sang Publishing Co., 1970.

Ja Hee. *The New Record.* Taipei: Chung Hwa Book Co., Ltd., 1981.

*Journal of Prenatal and Perinatal Psychology and Health, Vol. 14: 1 and 2.* Lawrence, KS: Allen Press, 1999.

Kim Do Hyang. *T'ae Gyo Umak.* Seoul: Seoul Audio Inc., 1992.

Kim Eun Joo. "Tradition Holds Sway for New Mothers." *Korean Identity.* Seoul: Yonhap News Agency, 1994.

Kushi, Michio and Aveline. *Macrobiotic Pregnancy and Care of the Newborn.* Tokyo: Japan Publications Inc., 1984.

Lee Bong Ju. *Story of Chong Mong-ju.* Seoul: So-dong Publishing Co., 1989.

Lee Won Sup. *The Royal Family's Teachings for Raising Life.* Seoul: Chorum, 1993.

_____. "Prenatal Care and Diet of Choson Royalty." August 7, 1999. *Korea Times.*

Legge, James. (trn.) *The She King, Vol. IV of The Chinese Classics*. Hong Kong: Hong Kong University Press, 1960.

Mattielli, Sandra. (ed.) *Virtues in Conflict*. "Boy Preference Reflected in Korean Folklore" by Cha Jae Ho, et al. Seoul: Royal Asiatic Society, 1977.

Oh Shi Rim. *Sim Sa Im Dang, and Child Education*. Seoul: Woo Sung Publishing Co., 1988.

Oshima Kyoshi. *T'ai Kyo*. Tokyo: Goma Books, 1988.

Seligson, Fred Jeremy. *Oriental Birth Dreams*. Seoul: Hollym Publishing Co., 1990.

Sung Woo Sok. *T'ae Gyo*. Seoul: Baek Yang Publishing Co., 1986.

Yo Sang Kek Kwa. "T'ae Gyo, 365 days." Seoul: *JAM JAM* (Woman's Magazine) August, 1990.

Zong Jo Chen. *Dr. Hsu Chi Tai's Principles for Women*. Taipei: 1983.